Mass Hysteria

Explorations in Bioethics and the Medical Humanities
Series Editor: James Lindemann Nelson

This series aims to include the most theoretically sophisticated, challenging, and original work being produced in the areas of bioethics, literature and medicine, law and medicine, philosophy of medicine, and history of medicine. *Explorations in Bioethics and the Medical Humanities* also features authoritative contributions to educational contexts and to public discourse on the meaning of health and health care in contemporary culture and on the difficult questions concerning the best directions for biomedicine to take in the future.

Mass Hysteria

Medicine, Culture, and Mothers' Bodies

Rebecca Kukla

ROWMAN & LITTLEFIELD PUBLISHERS, INC.
Lanham • Boulder • New York • Toronto • Oxford

ROWMAN & LITTLEFIELD PUBLISHERS, INC.

Published in the United States of America
by Rowman & Littlefield Publishers, Inc.
A wholly owned subsidary of The Rowman & Littlefield Publishing Group, Inc.
4501 Forbes Boulevard, Suite 200, Lanham, Maryland 20706
www.rowmanlittlefield.com

PO Box 317
Oxford
OX2 9RU, UK

British Library Cataloguing in Publication Information Available

Library of Congress Cataloging-in-Publication Data

Kukla, Rebecca, 1969-
  Mass hysteria : medicine, culture, and mothers' bodies / Rebecca Kukla.
      p. cm. — (Explorations in bioethics and the medical humanities)
  Includes bibliographical references and index.
  ISBN 0-7425-3357-3 (cloth : alk. paper) — ISBN 0-7425-3358-1 (pbk. : alk.
  paper)
  1. Pregnancy—Psychological aspects. 2. Pregnant women—Europe—History.
  3. Pregnant women—North America. 4. Pregnant women—Medical care. I.
  Title. II. Series.

  HQ1206.K785 2005
  618.2—dc22   2005012497

Printed in the United States of America

For Eli

Contents

List of Figures

Acknowledgments

Like most authors, I wrote this book while weaving in and out of various intellectual and social communities, each of which changed and challenged the path of my writing. As it happens, the four years it took me to complete this project also spanned several distinct phases of my life and several different homes in different parts of the world. I treasure the finished work as a witness to this complex narrative of shifting conversations, priorities, experiences, and places. It is more traditional to acknowledge the contributions of people and institutions than those of places and experiences. But I feel an intellectual debt of gratitude to my home in Ottawa; the tiny cliff-side Portuguese town of Azoia; the utopian haven of Victoria, British Columbia; and the unspeakably and unexpectedly welcoming city of Washington, DC, which took me in and nurtured me. And my two pregnancies—the first failed, the second resulting in the birth of my wonderful son—along with my experiences as a new mother directly provided the inspiration and the passion that created this work and saw it through to completion.

As for people, my most pressing debts are to two of my dear friends and most inspiring and generous intellectual compatriots, Sarah Hardy and Margaret O. Little. My editors, James Lindemann Nelson and Eve De Varo, were patient, helpful, and supportive. Conversations with Alisa Carse, Margueritte Deslauriers, Ruth Faden, Stephanie Irwin, Amy Mullin, Joseph Rouse, Leslie Smith, Karen Stohr, and Holly Taylor improved the book substantially. For intellectual and social companionship, support, and inspiration, I am grateful to the members of my working group on obstetrical risk management ("Science Driven, Woman Centered, Lawless")—Elizabeth Armstrong, Annie Drapkin

Lyerly, Miriam Kupperman, Lisa Mitchell, and again Maggie Little. The same goes for my fellow Greenwall Fellows at Johns Hopkins University—Gwynne Jenkins, Mark Greene, Naomi Seiler, Debra Matthews, Jon Tilbert, and Dan Larriviere. My prenatal class later developed into a well-established playgroup, and the members of this group provided a different but just as valuable form of support and inspiration during my first year as a mother, so special thanks are due to Nicole Meekin, Joanne Haché, Camille Bieman, Andrea Martinko, Michelle Copeland, and Tomoko Swenson and their lovely children. Audiences at Georgetown University, Trent University, and McGill University and at meetings of the Science and Literature Society, the Canadian Philosophical Association, and especially the Canadian Society for Women in Philosophy provided helpful comments and conversation.

This work was supported in part by the Greenwall Foundation, the Social Sciences and Humanities Research Council of Canada, the Phoebe R. Berman Bioethics Institute at Johns Hopkins University, and the philosophy departments at Carleton University and Georgetown University.

My parents, André Kukla and Kaila Kukla, and my sister, Elisa Kukla, have given me a lifelong commitment to love, family, and the pursuit of truth, justice, and the perfect turn of phrase. Last on this list but always closest to my heart, I owe the deepest gratitude to my husband, Richard, and my son, Eli, who provided love, inspiration, faith, fun, thought, meaning, time, and a room of my own.

PART
I

1

Introduction:
Impressionable Bodies

Female bodies, and especially pregnant and newly maternal bodies, leak, drip, squirt, expand, contract, crave, divide, sag, dilate, and expel. It is hard not to see why such bodies have long seemed to have dubious, hard to fix, permeable boundaries. And to the extent that we take the integrity and boundaries of the body as integrally intertwined with the integrity and boundaries of the self—and we have done so, at least throughout the history of Western culture and probably beyond—these dubious boundaries have been a source of various species of intellectual and visceral anxiety.[1] The maternal body has long been seen as posing a troubling counterpoint to the mythical well-bounded, fully unified, seamless masculine body.[2] At the same time, the capacity of the maternal body to nurture, via its womb and its breasts, seems to give its boundaries a different kind of lack of fixity: we imagine the maternal body as an 'organic unity' able to bridge the gap between two bodies, becoming both one and two at once through the gifts of gestation and milk. Thus the boundaries of the maternal body are unstable in these two different ways, which have been given different sets of meanings and normative valences over the years; both species of instability have captured our cultural imagination in multifaceted ways.

In this book, I want to look at how maternal and infant bodies are cared for within our medical and cultural institutions. I will argue for a mutually constitutive relationship between the dynamic boundaries of maternal bodies and the care these bodies have received. In caring for bodies, we mold them and change them in ways both subtle and dramatic. Imaginatively, we put bodies to use as symbols, and our ways of imagining and representing bodies have ethical, political, practical, and medical repercussions for those bodies. In turn our understanding of and anxieties over these boundaries give form to our standards for caring for them. I want to examine how we have tried to 'fix' the boundaries of mothers' bodies, imaginatively and in concrete practice, and equally how the lack of fixity of these boundaries has been imagined and understood and how it has impacted the social and medical status and treatment of these bodies. My interest in this work is specifically with *pregnant* bodies and the bodies of *new mothers with infants*—that is, bodies centrally defined by their maternality and reproductive function.[3]

Karen Barad has argued that the boundaries of the fetus as an object are not simply 'given' but are constituted through practiced 'boundary articulations,' including material practices of measuring and viewing fetuses and all the rituals that surround and embed such practices.[4] One needn't be any sort of radical social constructionist in order to notice and take seriously the fact that the fetus and, with it, the pregnant mother are not objects that come with ready-made stable boundaries. All romanticism and moral analysis aside, the maternal body incarnates one human at the beginning of pregnancy and two at the end of it, and it is by no means clear how to tell a coherent story of this passage. Debates around abortion issues have made the contestability of any such story clear. But upon reflection, we can see that we need not be worried about when it is or is not acceptable to terminate a pregnancy, nor with pinning down a crisp moment at which the fetus transforms into a person, in order to notice that the story of this passage from one to two is a complex and murky story to discern, involving negotiations of boundaries around and within persons that are contestable at each stage. Furthermore—and this is one of the substantive claims of this book—this story is one that is essentially mediated and given its shape by the social rituals and practices that make up pregnancy and motherhood, along with the representations and knowledge techniques that expectant and new mothers use to understand their own identities and boundaries, those of their fetuses and children, and the substantive, complex, dynamic relationships between them.

To make such claims is not to commit oneself to any kind of social constructionism that says that fetuses aren't 'real' outside of social practices of representing them. Rather, it is to take seriously how the boundaries of these real objects (and, *a forteriori*, the boundaries of the maternal bodies that contain them) are concretely negotiated through our practices of interacting with, knowing, and representing them. Much of the literature on cultural analyses of fetal representations, especially the literature by cultural anthropologists, is quick to assert that such representations and techniques construct the 'reality' of the fetus.[5] I take claims about the 'construction' of fetal reality with a grain of salt; on the one hand, they strike me as problematically insouciant with respect to the robust determinacy of biological reality, and on the other hand, they are getting at a point that is surely right, concerning the real, material impact of our social practices of management and surveillance upon the boundaries and the character of fetuses and maternal bodies. In any case, in this book I am not concerned with the (ill-defined) meta-issue as to whether fetal or maternal bodies are 'socially constructed' or not, but with a more specific question that already takes the public, material reality of such bodies as given—namely *what kind* of (real, public) objects are these bodies, and how are expectant and new mothers' identities contoured by the nature of these bodies? I want to know how the materiality and boundaries of mothers, infants, and fetuses take on robust and distinct forms.

The unfixed boundaries of the female reproductive body have captured the medical imagination from the start: Hippocratic medicine treated the female body as structured around a *hodos*, which was an open route extending from the orifices of the head to the vagina.[6] At the same time, Hippocrates insisted that women's skin was spongy and porous, making it especially permeable, and making women in turn more susceptible to passions, less protected against corrupting ingestions, and more voracious in their sexuality.[7] Furthermore, Hippocrates and Plato both helped initiate a long tradition of understanding the womb as having appetites of its own, and hence as serving as an independent, a-rational force beckoning foreign substances to cross the boundaries of the female body.[8] Until at least the seventeenth century, medical lore cast the inside of the female reproductive body and the generative process it housed as deeply mysterious, unstable, and potentially dangerous. The uterus was thought capable not just of expanding and contracting (an ability which has long impressed) but also of wandering throughout the female body, causing disease and distress as it traveled. Hysteria, which was originally defined as the wandering of the womb, was thought distinctive in being able to mimic any other disease at all; this made it not only highly potent but also particularly wily and difficult to diagnose or rule out.[9] Hippocrates went so far as to let hysteria effectively take over the whole terrain of women's illness by claiming that the womb is the origin of all diseases in women.[10] With appetites and cravings of its own, and encased in a permeable skin, it was thought that the womb could be coaxed or repelled from various places in the body with sweet and foul scents.[11] Barbara Duden has argued at length that in the seventeenth and early eighteenth centuries, the inside of the female body was seen as a fluid space in which not only did organs move, shift, and travel but also bodily liquids such as milk, blood, pus, and bile were transformed into one another and could emerge from any orifice in any form.[12]

The powers of the womb were both awesome and dangerous, for while the womb, unlike any other piece of the human body, was able to generate and nurture the human form, it was also easily permeated and corrupted and capable, once corrupted, of creating monsters and deformation. These twin powers to form and to deform called for careful protection of the womb's purity, especially given that the pregnant body was imagined as especially permeable, with little resistance against outside forces and eminently crossable boundaries. Across history, we have worried about what pregnant women eat, breathe, drink, and absorb, and (more or less vividly at different moments in history) even with what they see, smell, wish, and imagine, insofar as all these ingestions risk polluting the space of the womb. Even stronger, we have worried that the pregnant body *craves*—that it is not merely passively prone to penetration, but that it in fact is the seat of capricious and forceful appetites that beckon foreign substances in.[13] The whole notion of a craving—so deeply linked in our imagination with pregnancy—is of not just any appetite but an appetite that is inherently irrational, unpredictable, forceful, and hard to control or deny. Concerns with the permeability of the maternal body and with its appetites and cravings have in turn been partnered with concerns about the potential for corruption of the pure space of the womb through ingestion and permeation across the boundaries of this body.

Despite the ongoing, reasonably constant themes of permeability, craving, purity, and corruption across our last 2,500 years of imagining female reproductive bodies, I will be arguing that the medical and cultural status of mothers' bodies went through a profound transformation during the second half of the eighteenth century—a transformation intimately linked to the triumph of Enlightenment ideology, modern science, and the formation of the modern, humanist democracy. And I will claim that the practices that govern maternal and infant bodies and their care and treatment in contemporary North America are in a deep sense continuous with those that took hold during the late eighteenth century. Many writers concerned with the ethics and cultural theory of contemporary reproduction focus on how new technologies and cultural trends (new reproductive technologies, prenatal testing, transformations in the family, etc.) are *changing* the central meanings and practices that constitute reproduction and reproductive bodies.[14] While there are surely all sorts of interesting and subtle ways in which this is so, I will be trying to reveal the deep *continuities* in our care of maternal bodies over the last 250 (and to some extent the last 2,500) years, and accordingly I will portray our contemporary understanding of maternality and maternal bodies as deeply *modernist* (as opposed to distinctively postmodernist).

My main focus then, historically speaking, will be on two eras: Part I of this book is concerned primarily with Europe during the latter half of the eighteenth century and the first half of the nineteenth century—in particular, the time from Rousseau's publication of *Emile* (1755) through the fallout from the Revolutionary era. Part II of this book is concerned primarily with contemporary—that is, roughly post-1985—North America. However, even though I am arguing that a substantial shift in the situation of the maternal body occurred during the late eighteenth century, which gave birth to our 'modern' understanding of mothers' bodies, I want to portray this as a shift *within* a set of ongoing concerns, anxieties, practices, and understandings that have governed the care of these bodies since the start of recorded medicine during the Hippocratic era. The meaning and care of the maternal body underwent (and was central to) a revolution during the late Enlightenment, but this was a revolution that intensified, ossified, and polarized themes that were already present in cultural and medical practices and imagery. For this reason, this first chapter will step back and try to present the medical and cultural history out of which the shifts in the eighteenth century sprung by briefly examining the situation of maternal bodies in Europe in the early modern era (roughly 1600–1750). I will admit up front that I am not a historian; I have not tried to mount a comprehensive or complete historical argument about the care and boundaries of maternal bodies. Rather, in the first half of this book I will use historical sources selectively in order to reveal trends, ideas, images, and practices that served as beginnings of important contemporary narratives about mothers' bodies and their place within medicine and culture.

A "PRIVATE LOOKING-GLASSE"

I want to begin in the seventeenth century, when a flood of tracts on gynecology, obstetrics, and midwifery, authored by physicians but designed for a relatively wide audience, hit the shelves. Several of these achieved quite a bit of prominence and influence, including in particular Jakob Rüff's *The Expert Midwife*; Jacques Guillemeau's *Child-Birth, or the Happy Delivery of Women*; François Mauriceau's *The Diseases of Women with Child and in Childbed*; the anonymous work *The English Midwife Enlarged* (apparently plagiarized from James Wolveridge); John Sadler's *The Sicke Woman's Private Looking-Glasse*; Paul Portal's *The Complete Practice of Men and Women Midwives, or*

the *True Manner of Assisting a Woman in Child-Bearing*; Pierre Dionis' *A General Treatise on Midwifery*; and Nicholas Culpeper's *Directory for Midwives*.[15] The precursor for this series was Eucharius
Rösslin's *Der Swangern Frawen und Hebamman Rosengarten* (*The
Pregnant Woman's and Midwife's Rosegarden*), which appeared well
ahead of its time in 1513 and was translated into English in 1540.

During the sixteenth and seventeenth centuries, myths of the mobile, unstable, chameleon-like insides of the female reproductive body
existed alongside very little in the way of direct empirical knowledge
of these insides. Dissections of pregnant bodies were very rare.
Nicholas Culpeper, the great bawdy popularizer of the topic of reproductive medicine, commented on this rarity in 1651, noting that few
had ever seen the inside of the womb; he remarked, "I myself saw one
woman opened that died in child-bed, not delivered, and that is more
by one than most." Direct physical examinations of women, pregnant
or otherwise, were considered indecent and were not standard medical
practice. For reasons of modesty, male physicians based their diag-
noses and treatment decisions for women on their patients' own verbal reports and on other external signs. Even writing about the 'private
parts' of women had to be handled with care and could quickly be interpreted as an assault on decency and modesty. Midwifery was an exclusively female profession, and male surgeons were called to the
scene only during childbirth emergencies when leisurely examinations were neither appropriate nor medically possible.

For these reasons, the inside of the female reproductive body was
poorly understood when these early medical texts on obstetrics
emerged. The basic physical changes that mark pregnancy, such as
changes in the color and texture of the vaginal mucous, would not be
medically recognized until the nineteenth century; self-reports of
'quickening,' rather than third-personally available symptoms, played
the largest role in diagnosing pregnancy in the seventeenth century.[16]
Despite their authoritative medical voice and their focus on the
process of pregnancy and birth, very few of these texts attempt any
drawings of fetuses in the womb, though they contain lots of drawings
of obstetrical tools and monstrous births. In the few drawings that do
portray fetuses, the womb is represented as a pure, unarticulated
empty space without a placenta, politely and modestly disembodied
with no trace of the woman who contains it (in contrast to later
eighteenth-century representations—see frontispiece), and the fetus is
represented with the proportions and demeanor of a regular infant, differing only in size across the different stages of gestation.[17] Furthermore,
these depictions were highly stylized and constructed according to
conventions based in representational tradition rather than empirical
contact (see figure 1.1).[18] According to Barbara Duden, one seventeenth-

century doctor who saw an aborted fetus of four months' gestation concluded that it had to be a monster because of its disproportionately large head.[19] Elaborate descriptions of fetal positions in the womb were derived from external signs and from experiences during childbirth, rather than from direct contact with the pregnant body.

Against the background of the privacy of the female body and the indecency and immodesty involved in displaying it to the public and/or masculine gaze or touch, these medical texts inhabit a challenging position with respect to voice and audience, and often these challenges are quite explicit. Most of the texts are explicitly addressed to women, and more specifically to women *patients*, with the goal of empowering them in their ability to get effective medical help. For instance John Sadler's *The Sicke Woman's Private Looking-Glasse*, whose title already betrays the unusual status of a text that is making the private public, puts in its subtitle that it exists for "enabling Women to informe the Physician about the cause of their grief," and it begins by decrying the suffering that has issued from women's "ignorance and modesty." Sadler argues that this ignorance and modesty produces ineffective obstetric patients.[20] The anonymous author of *The English Midwife Enlarged* negotiates his uncomfortable status as a male author writing on topics that are inappropriate for men by writing his text as a series of questions answered by a mythical female midwife, thereby—in a lovely inversion of convention—artificially *feminizing* the authoritative voice of the text.

Once we set this spate of books against their cultural background, in which man-midwifery was socially taboo for the most part and the female body was privatized and off limits, they emerge as not only requiring a creative negotiation of audience and voice but indeed as intrinsically political—even, one might claim with some anachronism, feminist. In addition to explicitly claiming the goal of empowering

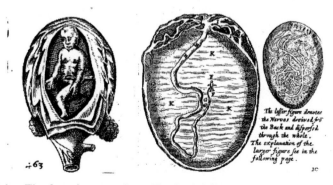

Figure 1.1.   The fetus in utero, from *The English Mid-wife Enlarged* (London: Rowland Reynolds, 1682), 10, 34, courtesy of the National Library of Medicine.

female patients and combating unnecessary female ignorance, they go out of their way to note that they risk offending modesty, and sometimes attack the codes of modesty and the taboos against man-midwifery that keep the female body off limits.[21] They often take pointed pleasure in discussing highly taboo topics such as venereal disease and female orgasms and sexual pleasures. Nicholas Culpeper, in particular, relished in his descriptions of the male 'yard' and the conditions under which women received pleasure from it; he introduces his section on female genitalia with the comment, "Having served my own sex, I shall now see if I can please the women, who have no more cause than men (that I know of) to be ashamed of what they have." Thus we need to read these works as as-yet-incomplete beginnings of a politicized transformation of the status and publicity of the maternal body, as patient and as medical object.

PERMEABLE AND PERAMBULATING WOMBS

In Jakob Rüff's sixteenth-century textbook *The Expert Midwife*, we learn that the fetus

> Is most like a tender flower and blossom of trees, which is easily cast down and dejected with any blast of wind and rain, and for that cause there is neede of very great caution and heed to be taken, that no peril and danger may happen to them that are with childe by any manner of means, either by sudden fear, affrightments, by fire, lightning, thunder, with monstrous and hideous aspects and sights of men and beasts, by immoderate joy, sorrow and lamentation; or by untemperate motion and exercise of running, leaping, riding, or by surfeit or repletion by meate and drinke; or that they being taken with any disease do not use sharp and violent medicines using the counsel of unskillfull physicians.

This vivid imagery of the fetus as a fragile and ill-protected being inhabiting a dangerous space within the maternal body, and the latter as in turn needing detailed and extensive protection and regulation, is emblematic of a pervasive and potent vision of the nature of pregnancy and the space it provides—one that was especially explicit during the seventeenth century and in the medical texts of the time.

The seventeenth-century textbooks are particularly concerned about and often organized around the possibility of deformed births, with a special focus on the dangers of the impure, permeated womb. Sadler's book, for instance, is organized primarily as a list of ways in which the womb can fail to maintain its purity and its integrity—the womb here leaks and 'weeps,' and various 'corrupt humours' flow in and out of it, making nothing more 'perilous' to the body than the 'ill-affected womb.' Many of the works go into elaborate detail, describing and often visually representing famous cases of monstrous births.[22] Monstrous births could be the product of weak seed or impure blood, of conception during menstruation, of the woman fertilizing herself with her own seed (!), or, most importantly and consistently, of maternal ingestions of sights and substances that could pollute or deform the womb. In justifying the need for careful knowledge and monitoring of the maternal body, in the preface of his book, Sadler warns us: "From the womb come convulsions, epilepsies, apoplexies, palseys, hecticke fevers, dropsies, malignant ulcers, and to bee short, there is no disease so ill but may proceed from the evil quality of it."

In these works, there is no sense that normal, healthy birth is the routine outcome of pregnancy (which it wasn't). Instead, pregnancies and births are divided into the false and the true (usually interpreted as a distinction between 'moles,' or unarticulated growths in the womb, and formed fetuses) and the monstrous and the nonmonstrous, with both possibilities in each case being equally plausible pregnancy outcomes. Mauquest de la Motte wrote that "a woman that has certain signs of being with child ought to be careful, and do all she can to bring to the full time; she must not put her confidence in her strength, youth, or good constitution, but on the contrary must look upon a big belly as a disease, which she ought to have a watchful eye over."[23] Pregnancy was a dangerous process akin to a disease rather than one that would generally unfold in an orderly fashion if left to its own devices, and the maternal body was an untrustworthy entity requiring careful surveillance even when it appeared strong and well-ordered.

Mary Fissell[24] has argued that the emergence of this new genre of midwifery and obstetrical texts was coincident with—and partly constitutive of—a new level of concern with the potential of the female reproductive body to be corrupted and corrupting. The mother's potential ingestions—of food, drink, drugs, but also sights and other experiences causing immoderate passions—were particularly targeted as a source of corruption of the fragile fetus. Indeed, the dangers of the impurity of the maternal body and its corrupting possibilities outstripped pregnancy and applied to new motherhood as well, for as Culpeper commented, "If the blood be impure . . . then it is not fitting that a woman should give her child suck very speedily after her delivery; for if the blood be impure, how can it breed good milk? Dirty water will make but dirty porrage."[25] Milk was seen as a direct medium of transference of the nature of the nursing body, not only physical but moral, to the infant. As Jacques Guillemeau put it, "The child that sucks an nurse, that is vitious, and wicked, sucks also from her, her faults and vices."[26]

The perceived special threat of the pollution of the womb has its ground in twin, intertwined tropes in the imagination of the space of the maternal body. On the one hand, the boundaries of the maternal body could not be trusted to protect this space, both because of the permeability and instability of these boundaries and because of expectant mothers' own untrustworthy propensity to crave—for everyone recognized pregnant women's "strange and deprav'd appetite for uncommon things,"[27] although experts disagreed as to whether these depravities needed to be indulged (as Dionis argued) or policed (as was maintained by Rüff and Sadler). The maternal body was thus especially prone to irrational ingestions, and these ingestions translated themselves especially directly to the womb, for as Jane Sharp put it, in the first midwifery text written by a British woman, "the womb partakes" of whatever impresses itself upon us, for "the womb is affected as our senses are."[28]

On the other hand, the womb itself, during this period, was seen as the seat not only of affectation but also of its own appetites, and indeed as a busy little organ that communicated with the rest of the body and contributed actively to the form of the fetus. Although Aristotelians conceived of the womb as a passive environment for the fetus, whose form is determined in advance, this tradition was mostly out of favor in seventeenth-century medical circles. Sadler refers to the womb routinely as an 'agent' in contrast with the blood and seed that provide the 'matter' of pregnancy. In response to James Blondel's *Strength of Imagination in Pregnant Woman Examined*,[29] Daniel Turner[30] mocks those few authors, including Blondel, who do not believe in the control exercised by the womb over the form of the fetus, as 'paralyzing' the womb and treating it as a 'paralytic man.' Guillaume Mauquest de la Motte[31] took sides in the debate over the uterus's active role in fetal development by citing its 'wonderful' ability to dilate and contract and its ability to 'answer to the intention of nature.' Culpeper, characteristically, takes women's active sexual drive and clitoral orgasm as essential to conception and uses them as a premise from which to infer that the female body must play an active role in fetal formation as well. This metonymic association between sexual appetite and the active role of the uterus in conception is common: Dionis writes, "In these favorable and happy circumstances, the Yard being erected, and introduced into the Vagina, the Seed immited directly into the mouth of the Womb, is *greedily* receiv'd, and by the contraction of the Uterus, is pushed through the Tube Fallopiane." This association between sexual appetite and the activity of the womb is an interestingly double-edged phenomenon: on the one hand it lies at the center of what was clearly a progressive valuing of women's independent sexual pleasures, described in appreciative detail in defiance of the mores of the time, while at the very same time these same, linked appetitive dimensions of the maternal body are feared as potential sources of monstrosity and disorder. For instance Rüff cites the 'attractive vertue' of the uterus itself as an explanation for bestial conceptions resulting in monstrous births; here the inner cravings of the womb become forces of attraction (to the bestial seed?), which themselves drive the sexual appetites of the woman who houses them. It is precisely in *empowering* the female body as an appetitive agent that these authors vividly call forth the specter of appetites and agency gone wrong, subverting rather than enabling proper, natural form.

THE MATERNAL IMAGINATION

According to most of the authors of the sixteenth through early eighteenth centuries, an expectant mother's cravings, desires, and experiences—especially experiences that aroused strong passions such as fear and lust—were capable of *directly* inscribing themselves upon the body of the fetus, producing deformities and monstrosities that retained the semantic content of the original impression. The theory that this kind of transference was possible—regularly referred to as the "theory of the maternal imagination"—is an especially fertile, vivid, and historically important site for the medical concerns with the transparency and permeability of the maternal body and the corresponding threat of a corrupted and corrupting womb. First of all, the theory of the maternal imagination is a particularly dramatic example of the idea that the boundaries of the maternal body have a distinctive kind of transparency or permeability to them, calling for special protective measures. Second, the fact that according to this theory, fetal bodies are impacted by the mother's activities, not just *causally* but in a way that in an important sense maintains the *meaning* or intentional content of the mother's behavior, brings to life the idea that reproductive processes are somehow infused with *agency*—it is the mother's *intentional states* that here build (or pervert) the form of the fetal body. Finally, the scope of the impact of maternal imagination upon pregnancy was a hotly contested and imaginatively engaging topic within the medical discourse of the time.

The theory of the maternal imagination again has ancient origins, and it has resurfaced over the centuries. As recently as the 1930s, a state-produced pregnancy manual felt it important to assure mothers that "very few babies have birthmarks and yet most women at some time during the nine months of pregnancy see some of the unpleasant or startling things that tradition says will 'mark' your babies. So no mother need worry about 'marking' her baby. . . . There is no connection between [the birthmark] and anything the mother has seen or done."[32] However, the theory certainly had its medical heyday in the sixteenth and seventeenth centuries, where pretty much every medical text included a discussion of it. This was no folk theory, during this era, but rather a topic for the most scientifically minded members of the medical community (prominently including Malebranche, among others), who offered physicalist 'explanations' of the phenomenon and indeed often set themselves dialectically against purportedly backward, anti-scientific, religious types who believed in fetal preformation and in the inertness of the female body. Rüff, for instance, sets up the debate over the maternal imagination as one of whether monsters are caused by 'judgments of God' or by the much more mundane 'corruption of seed.' He comes down on the latter side, with the claim that "through longings and terrors, many are born, which have diverse spots and marks imprinted on the body."

It is *frights, cravings,* and *sexual arousals* that are by far the most often cited passions attributed with marking the fetus. Some of the most common claims were that cravings for strawberries and other fruits caused birthmarks resembling those fruits; cravings for shellfish caused particularly grotesque facial deformities; fright by a bear would cause a hairy child; being startled by a hare would cause a harelip, or cleft palate; and lascivious thoughts could produce hermaphrodism and other obscene monstrosities. Frights in the mother could wound the skin of the child, and limbs could be mutilated and truncated by the sight of a 'mendicant' with no arms.[33] Hence it is not any old strong passions or imaginative representations, but in particular those bound up with maternal *appetites* (be they attractive or repulsive) that are the real risks. Here again, we see that women's cravings—their tendencies to draw things in and repel things across the boundaries of their bodies—are a particular source of concern. Indeed, for Turner, the appetite is explicitly the mechanism that transfers the effect from maternal environment to fetus: "The fancy, once excited at the Appearance of the Object, presently stirs up the Appetite, and this latter, local motion, by which to approach or shun the said object." This combination of maternal permeability and maternal appetite is, as we have already seen, cause for medical anxieties over the purity of the fetal environment.

This cluster of anxieties is sometimes intertwined with other familiar social anxieties that circulate around reproduction. In a fascinating twist, Sadler warns that the child of an adulteress may still look like her husband because she may have been thinking about him guiltily during coitus. In this case, anxieties around how paternity can be secured intersect with anxieties about the maternal imagination, through the warning that fathers cannot even trust family resemblance as a marker of proper paternity. This example doubles the call to carefully police women's appetites: her wayward cravings may betray her husband and her child at once. Sadler also cites a commonly mentioned report of a woman who "conceived and brought forth an Etheopian" because she looked at a painting of a black man during conception, thereby adding anxieties surrounding racial purity to the mix of concerns.[34] Women's cravings and imagination can thus deform and denature both the kinship order and the racial order, along with the order of their children's bodies, in ways that normal, external controls over sexual activity cannot prevent.

During this era, throughout which the female body was more or less cloaked in modesty and obscurity, the theory of the maternal imagination granted the female reproductive body a useful and powerful kind of transparency. Though no one could see into the womb, the resulting child could be 'read' as a kind of biography of the mother's activities and (especially) private passions and cravings during pregnancy. The infant body served as a testimony and tribunal of the mother's wayward wandering and appetites. And in fact, the transparency was double, for the sights that stimulated the maternal imagination could be transferred without distortion or loss of meaning, across the mother's skin and uterine wall, and onto the body of the infant.

Indeed, the immediacy and transparency of the connection between mother and fetus was part of what was at stake in the debates over the force of the maternal imagination. James Blondel, an opponent of the theory of the maternal imagination, claims that "the mother and the child in utero are no more related than when it is feeding on the nurse's knee or playing in the cradle," and "the child is as distinct from the mother as a child at the breast, separate from its nurse upon which it feeds, and it is no more possible for the mother's imagination to act upon the child in utero, than for the nurse to make by her fancy, upon the suckling baby, any mark or impression."[35] Daniel Turner, for his part, not only disagrees with Blondel's assertion of separateness in the course of his defense of the force of the maternal imagination but also clearly finds it nearly indecent—he reinscribes this same quotation over and over again, and his shock at its absurdity forms the rhetorical centerpiece of his book. In turn, the book reads as a polemic on the fundamental oneness of mother and fetus as much as it does a defense of the theory of the maternal imagination itself.

Given that the actual anatomy and mechanical workings of the reproductive body were not well understood, it would have been hard to come up with good causal stories about the effect of various maternal environments and activities on fetal development. In this respect, the theory of the maternal imagination was a useful medical tool. It provided the basis for a technic for protecting healthy fetal development, which drew upon meaningful and symbolic—rather than causal and mechanistic—relationships between the external life of the gestating woman and the internal growth of her fetus. The medical texts of the time are filled with advice for doctors, midwives, husbands, and expectant mothers concerning which activities, sights, and experiences the mother should avoid in order to prevent marking or deforming her baby via her imaginative passions and appetites. Culpeper writes succinctly, "And though doctors cannot cure monsters, yet they are to admonish women with child not to look upon monsters." The transmission of meanings and ideas from the external world onto the bodies of infants bypasses the need to work out a causal theory of fetal impact, for the potential deformities and the means for avoiding them can be hermeneutically 'read' rather than causally explained. As Turner puts it, the mother's imagination does not causally impact the fetal body so much as it produces 'signatures' upon this body. It is no surprise that scientific enthusiasm for the theory of the maternal imagination would drop precipitously in the late eighteenth century, when the female reproductive body did become genuinely public and medicalized, and its anatomical features and causal propensities were more or less properly understood.[36]

There is a tension here that needs to be explored, for as I pointed out, the defenders of the theory of the maternal imagination were very much invested in coming up with a naturalist understanding and discourse of pregnancy, rather than one relying upon divine or supernatural forces; they saw themselves as bringing the pregnant body into the domain of science. But naturalistic science traditionally deals in causes, not in sympathies and symbolism, and in fact it was just this causal, mechanistic vision of science that captured the seventeenth-century imagination. The whole symbolic, semiotic form of the maternal imagination seems to sit badly with this naturalistic agenda. Indeed, most of the defenders of the maternal imagination made some attempt to use vaguely causal language to explain the phenomenon, referring to the 'delicacy of the nerves' or other ill-defined anatomical reasons why maternal bodies would be especially able to transmit intact experiences from outside to inside.

In order to understand what was at stake here, we need to remember the role that the passions played in seventeenth-century natural philosophy. Passions and appetites inhabited an interesting border territory between the realm of the mental and meaningful and the realm of the bodily and brutely causal. They had intentional objects—that is, they were *about* something—but they were different from traditional mental states such as beliefs. Beliefs could be considered dispassionately and were governed by rational manipulation. Passions, on the other hand, were subject to the capricious logic of the body, and the agent could not spontaneously control them but was rather passively subject to them (as their name implies), and they were appetitive rather than just reflective of reality. Passions, despite their meaningful content, traded in and operated through somatic urges and responses rather than the cold, dispassionate light of reason. Thus the passions provided the perfect medium for meanings to translate themselves from the world onto bodies. Women's pregnant bodies, with their weaker resistance to passions and their intense cravings, their higher impressionability, and the fragile or nonexistent boundaries separating them from their fetuses, were in turn 'natural' sites for such passionate transmissions.

By bringing meanings into the domain of the body's naturalistic processes and making them fair game for physicians' scrutiny, diagnosis, and medical management, the theory of the maternal imagination forges a crucial link between medical obstetrics and the management of maternal character and ethics—a link that, we will see, far outlasts the theory itself. According to the theory, mothers' passions, experiences, and especially appetites are directly relevant to fetal outcome, and fetal bodies can be read as testimony of them. But passions, experiences, and appetites are critical to character and are normatively assessable in a way that brutely physical features are not. Furthermore, they are *private*—even though they may be publicly revealed after the fact by the child they mark, medical examination cannot uncover them. They are also transitory rather than stable features of maternal bodies—thoughts, experiences, and appetites shift moment by moment. Thus these medically potent, inner states cannot be directly seen or even stably diagnosed. Instead, physicians and husbands needed to control for them indirectly, by making sure that expectant mothers had the strength of character to withstand inappropriate passions and appetites and the ethical conduct to avoid behavior leading to inappropriate experiences. And this was a strenuous task, for remember that passions and appetites alone were thought sufficient to mark the child, whether or not the mother actually gave in to or acted upon them (much as we now hear about how maternal stress and anger during pregnancy may somehow damage the fetus).

Maternal impressions could be activated by such a wide range of objects—from portraits to animals to members of other races and onward—that almost no dimension of a pregnant woman's life was truly safe. Doctors could do little to control pregnant women's inner lives. All they could do was warn expectant parents about the obstetrical significance of women's character and ethical fiber and, when relevant, use the deformed fetus as ex post facto testimony to her wayward or weak nature—and indeed, the texts of the time are rife with descriptions of how monstrous births betrayed the untoward temptations, activities, and proclivities of their mothers.[37] They could, on the other hand, recommend external restrictions or 'confinements' for pregnant women, which would reduce the chances of their having dangerous experiences. There were volumes of both 'expert' and folk knowledge circulating on how best to confine and domesticate the environment of expectant mothers in order to avoid the possibility of monstrous births.[38] Pregnant women needed protection in the form of a mostly sanitized, unstimulating, unsurprising environment. Obstetrical care required the ethical and practical regulation of women's activities, but not much by way of examinations and interventions into her body.

It is too simple to read the theory of the maternal imagination just as a tool for controlling women's mobility and policing their character.[39] We have seen that the theory also lay at the center of a move to attribute an important kind of agency to women's bodies, rather than treating them as merely subject to the will of God or as passive sites for the development of male seed. Likewise, the theory partook in a movement toward giving women the informational tools to help control their medical destiny, as many of these manuals make explicit. On the one hand, then, this movement was liberating insofar as it granted agency and responsibility to female obstetrical patients and to the interventions of science, rather than treating fetal outcomes as the products of God's will and obstetrical patients as passive subjects with no need for medical knowledge and no need to participate in their own health care. On the other hand, the theory of the maternal imagination, and other beliefs about the potential of the maternal body to corrupt the space of the womb and the fetal form, inextricably linked maternal ethics and character with medical concerns about birth outcomes. Birth outcomes were testimonies to maternal character and vice, with all of the space for blame, recrimination, and the general moralizing of medicine that this brought with it. Through personal responsibility and well-regulated character, women could help control these outcomes, and through proper medical education women could become more effective patients. Both prongs of this movement have in fact lasted and continue to permeate contemporary obstetrical practices and rhetoric: contemporary pregnant women are expected to be avid consumers of medical information, to actively participate in their own prenatal care, and to aggressively pursue good birth outcomes, while these outcomes are cast as testimony to individual maternal character.[40]

Despite the link between personal character and pregnancy outcomes that the theory of the maternal imagination forged, these seventeenth-century texts treated monstrous births, and the maternal vices, weaknesses, and missteps they might reveal, as fundamentally *private* matters. There is no particular sense, in these early obstetrical texts, that a monstrous birth has any civic or social significance, nor, in particular, that it is society's job to be invested in pregnancy outcomes or to police maternal character and activities. *Doctors* and midwives are concerned with monstrous births as *medical* problems, and hence maternal passions and actions are their business, and these texts take it for granted, reasonably enough, that expectant *mothers* (and sometimes fathers) have a strong personal stake in avoiding monstrous births and producing healthy, well-formed children. But the medical texts were remarkably free of any political rhetoric about the social burden of monstrous births or the civic importance of producing healthy babies, and also of any larger judgmental rhetoric concerning maternal vice, beyond blaming it for poor fetal outcome. It is clear that the birth of a deformed child produced much tongue-wagging and 'tsk-tsk'-ing in the community.[41] Such births also made for good yarns with obvious sensationalist appeal in the medical literature. Yet no one seemed to see the births as a social problem, but more as a personal burden and embarrassment for the family. This may largely reflect facts about the structure of society, including its lack of large-scale social welfare and support networks—but it is hard to confidently interpret silences. For the moment, I just want to set the stage for the changes to come by pointing out that the texts of the time refrained from attaching social or moral meanings to maternal activities and fetal outcomes beyond the very local meanings specific to a particular birth.

GOVERNING AND ORDERING MATERNAL BODIES

A recurring theme in almost all of these early modern medical texts on pregnancy and human reproduction is that the pregnant body (along with the fetal body, and to a lesser extent, the infant body) is not simply a given, static entity with a fixed 'nature,' but rather a dynamic entity that needs to be *governed* and *ordered*. This governing and ordering of the maternal body was portrayed as a joint task of physicians, who prescribed bodily routines, and expectant mothers, who were positioned as responsible for elaborate routines of bodily self-management. A whole series of book and chapter titles of the time reinscribe this idea that the *bodies themselves* are proper objects of government and ordering. Culpeper has chapters entitled "The Governance of Woman with Child" and "The Governance of Woman in Child-Bed," as well as "How a woman that would have children should order her body." Mauriceau has a chapter called "Of the diet and ordering of a new-born Babe," and Guillemeau's *Childbirth, or the Happy Delivery of Women*, is subtitled "wherein is set downe the government of women." His book, too, attributes responsibility for this project of governance to doctors and women alike, with chapters entitled "The governing and ordering of a woman, the nine months she goes with child" and "How a woman must govern her selfe all the time of her being with child." William Sermon's sermon-length book title is *The Ladies' companion, or the English Midwife, wherein is demonstrated the manner and order how women ought to govern themselves during the whole times of their breeding children and of their difficult labour, hard travail, and lying-in, etc., together with the diseases they are subject to (especially in such times) and the several wayes and means to help them; also the various forms of the child's proceeding forth of the womb, in 17 copper cuts, with a discourse of the parts principally serving for generation.*[42] Each of these texts contains elaborate rules for the active management of the body: precise rules concerning diet, exercise, clothing, tonics, amount of exposure to the outdoors, and sexual activity as well as precise rituals and recipes for caring for the breasts, skin, and other body parts, not to mention, of course, rules for avoiding the inappropriate incitement of the passions, which included mental exercises as well as restrictions of environment. They also prescribe the diet, sleeping positions, clothing, sleep schedule, etc., of infants.

Several features of these prescriptive discussions are interesting. First of all, they clearly take the pregnant body as one whose very nature can and should be subject to active shaping. As if foreshadowing Foucaultian jargon and sensibilities, the rhetoric of ordering the *body* or the *woman* here is insistent and startling: these texts do not call just for the governing of *behavior* or even the passions but, quite clearly, of the material body itself. If we stereotype the early modern era as one in which inert, mechanistically deterministic nature was opposed to the normative domain of the intellect, this language should surprise us. The pregnant body was not a given entity with a fixed nature but one whose nature could be shaped and regulated. A pregnancy was considered 'unnatural' when it was nonstandard or disorderly, either because of the position of the fetus in the womb, or because of a deformation or lack of formation in the fetus itself. There was nothing strange about *helping* a pregnancy to be natural, by governing the body to help produce a well-formed child or manipulating the body to position the fetus correctly in the womb. Only later would 'natural' pregnancy and childbirth come to be associated with freedom from artificial manipulations and interventions.

It is striking, also, the extent to which pregnancy is portrayed in these texts not as a passive state but as an active project requiring self-discipline and work on the part of expectant mothers, who, under these regimes of ordering and governing, were not merely *subjected to* various medical interventions but asked to *work at* their own pregnancies through disciplining their diet, doing various exercises, changing their practices of bathing and drinking, and so forth. Some feminist writing on pregnancy has tended to stereotype the male medical establishment as invested in treating women, and women's bodies, as passive objects for their manipulations and interventions and as passive sites of the natural unfolding of pregnancy.[43] Other sources—especially those connected with the modern midwifery community—have idealized earlier times as those in which pregnancy was treated as a 'natural' process in the sense of one to be left to unfold according to its own internal plans and order.[44] However, these texts belie both of these simplistic historical myths. In particular, as the reproductive female body was right on the brink of becoming a genuine, institutionalized medical object, the male doctors who were in the midst of negotiating this transition had a quite different view of pregnancy. They portrayed the pregnant body as a whole, and the womb within it, as active and malleable, and pregnancy as a project requiring proper discipline, not only from external medical forces but also from the pregnant woman herself; this picture in fact went hand in hand with the belief that the fetal form was not predestined but instead subject to maternal influence. We can reasonably view these requirements either as empowering, noticing how these authors attributed agency and responsibility to pregnant bodies, or as oppressive, noticing the stringent demands placed on the pregnant body and the basic distrust of its functioning and of women's capacities to control themselves and to effectively police their own boundaries and appetites.

We have seen that according to seventeenth-century medical writers, fetal outcomes could be damaged by any number of failures in the management of the maternal body. The space of the womb could be penetrated by the wrong passions, food, drink, bodily fluids, or medicines, or it could stray from its proper position and arrangement according to its own appetites. The volatile, penetrable, unstably bounded space of the maternal body was thus an untrustworthy site for the generation of new persons. Accordingly, the responsible, informed pregnant woman, empowered by medical knowledge, would govern and order her body with the help of medical professionals, participating actively in the project of protecting the health and well-formed nature of her future child.

In the seventeenth century, very few women were literate, and the experiences of pregnancy and childbirth were not considered a decent topic for public conversation. Hence it is not surprising that there is little documentation of how women in this era internalized these pictures of the dangers and the possibilities of their own bodies. We do not know much about how the theory of the maternal imagination and the threat of monstrous births permeated the phenomenology of pregnancy, or how they shaped women's lived sense of their own maternal responsibilities. Barbara Duden claims to take up exactly this question in her work *The Woman Beneath the Skin*;[45] it is ironic, therefore, that her source is the diary of a seventeenth-century *physician* who took notes on his own second-personal encounters with his female patients. In part II of this book, I will devote a lot of time to trying to uncover the phenomenology of pregnancy and early motherhood, in the context of contemporary North American culture. In the meantime, we can only imagine how these seventeenth-century textbooks, which were explicitly written in a second-person voice for women's consumption, might have impacted women's first-personal experiences of their own bodies and births.

PRESERVING NATURE

In a crucial and specific sense, the seventeenth-century goals for birth outcomes were modest. We have seen how the warnings and anxieties surrounding the possibility that the maternal body may corrupt or deform its infant show that in this era, fetal nature was not seen as stable and given but as malleable and subject to the influence of maternal activities and pollution via the permeation of maternal boundaries. But amidst all of these warnings, not once does any author raise the possibility that maternal activities or the protection of maternal boundaries might *enhance* the quality of a fetus, improving its nature beyond the benchmark of nondeformity and noncorruption. The wrong maternal passions could produce monsters, but there is no legacy, from this era, of thinking that the *right* maternal passions could improve the virtue, health, or form of the fetus beyond what it would attain if it merely remained uninfluenced and uncorrupted. Similarly, the many recommendations for 'ordering' and 'governing' the maternal body all aim at producing an infant who has not been *harmed* or *corrupted* by the mother. The goal was to avoid "monsters, mixed-breeds, marks and mutilations," as Turner puts it. Indeed, this picture of natural form as one to be preserved or deformed but not enhanced is implicit in the representations of the fetus we saw earlier: if the fetus already has a more-or-less complete adult form at each stage of development, presumably the job of the maternal body is to protect rather than develop this form along the way.

Thus even though these authors took maternal bodies as agents that played an active role in determining fetal nature, the goal in the medical governance of these bodies was to *eliminate* this influence, to *protect* the space of the womb from pollution, and likewise to keep the womb *pure*. Although nature is malleable, its best and most proper work will be done when external influences are minimized. Culpeper writes that as long as the womb is kept "pure," then "nature, having pure matter to work on, may make her work perfect, and so subject to live and not prone to die." This passage not only expresses a distinct conception of nature, as pollutable and deformable but not improvable, but also makes vivid the relatively low standards of the time for fetal 'perfection,' namely robust viability—more or less just *not dying*. Given the high infant mortality rates of the time,[46] this was a sufficiently lofty goal. 'Natural' fetal form was taken as a *benchmark* to be achieved but not surpassed. It serves as a nonnegotiable normative tribunal of proper form. This conception displays an interestingly double-edged picture of *given* nature as at once malleable, up to a point, and also setting its own fixed, independent constraints upon the limits of human intervention and purposiveness.

In this regard, our medical rhetoric and goals have changed rather markedly over the centuries. We still worry deeply about maternal ingestions and permeability, the pollution of the womb, and the possibility of deformed births, and we still demand rigorous regimens of self-management from pregnant women.[47] But our goal, now, tends to be more than mere viability: we aim to *improve* and hone fetal nature beyond what it would reach if left to its own devices—we recommend all sorts of elaborate practices for pregnant women, from simple folic acid supplements to piping Mozart into the womb, that are designed to utilize the permeability and impressionability of the maternal body toward the end of improving and perfecting fetal nature well beyond the benchmark of nonintervention and viability. As Elizabeth Armstrong puts it, we have shifted attention from the 'quantity' to the 'quality' of children.[48] I will argue in the next two chapters that our understanding of human nature was importantly transformed in the latter half of the eighteenth century, engendering conceptions of nature as indefinitely improvable and of maternal bodies as having the potential to enhance as well as to deform and pollute the bodies of their progeny.

But in these seventeenth-century texts, there is no trace of the rhetoric of enhancement. I found such enhancement mentioned as a possibility only once, as a *reductio* in an argument against the theory of the maternal imagination. Giovanni Bianchini, one of theory's most prominent detractors, writes,

> Were the form of the foetus in the power of the imagination, our offspring would be as subject to the capriciousness of mankind as our clothes. The form of the child's mouth, nose, eye, eyebrow, or any of its features, would as much depend on the reigning fashion, as the cut of a cap, coat, or any part of our dress.[49]

Here, the idea that babies could be 'designed' and not just protected from deformity and disease is taken as a fantasy, providing sufficient reason to reject any proposed causal mechanism that might make it plausible. It is not hard to notice that this vision of the designed baby is now very much on the table as a medical possibility and a cultural vision of how ideal gestation might proceed. Those horrified rather than compelled by this vision now tend to have ethical rather than scientific objections to it; indeed, we now generally treat our potentially indefinite ability to design and improve fetal bodies as a scientific inevitability, though our actual scientific advances so far do not justify this limitless confidence.[50] Contemporary commentators often suggest that 'designer babies' are a postmodern possibility put on the table by very recent technological advances. I will try to show that, on the contrary, this idea that we can design and perfect human nature through the work of the maternal body in fact had its primary birthplace in late-eighteenth-century France.

NOTES

1. Susan Bordo, in her classic book *Unbearable Weight: Feminism, Western Culture and the Body* (Berkeley: University of California Press, 1995), has done an excellent and oft-cited job of examining this type of concern with the integrity and boundaries of bodies and selves. I do not much care, here, if this concern with the vagaries of the bound-

aries of bodies in general, and female reproductive bodies in particular, is a universal dimension of 'human nature' or whether it is culturally inculcated but very widespread; it seems to me likely to have as much of a claim to being an inescapable product of the human condition as anything does.

2. In *Existentialism and Human Emotions* (New York: Philosophical Library, 1957), Jean-Paul Sartre argues that the fundamental, ego-structuring human/male trauma is the recognition that the body has holes and hollow spaces.

3. I will be spending much less time, I should note, on laboring bodies. Childbirth interests me less than pregnancy and early motherhood. This is mostly because my major interest and investment is in practices that make up the *ongoing, daily life and care* of mothers. The event of labor is almost surreally severed from the narrative of the rest of life both before and after—a phenomenon that would be worth exploring in its own right, which I suspect is integrally linked to why women have a hard time remembering their own labor. Labor forms a discrete, dramatic *event* rather than an ongoing *identity* or project. Many of us spend part of our lives *being pregnant* and *being mothers of infants*—for most of us, these become defining and extended projects with deep formative effects on our ongoing identities and on the rest of our projects. Pregnancy and early motherhood are thus open to a rich ethical and political texture as phenomena that I don't believe birth has, for all its excitement and its medical importance. Amy Mullin has given an interestingly similar justification for mostly skipping birth in order to focus on pregnancy and motherhood in *Reconceiving Pregnancy and Childcare* (New York: Cambridge University Press, 2005).

4. Karen Barad, "Getting Real: Technoscientific Practices and the Materialization of Reality," *Differences* 10(2), 1998, 86–128; see especially 115.

5. See for example Lorna Weir, "Pregnancy Ultrasound in Maternal Discourse," in *Vital Signs*, ed. Margrit Shildrick and Janet Price (Edinburgh: Edinburgh University Press, 1998) 78–101; Karen Newman, *Fetal Positions* (Palo Alto: Stanford University Press, 1996); Rayna Rapp, *Testing Women, Testing the Fetus* (New York: Routledge, 1999); and Rosalind Pollack Petchesky, "Fetal Images," *Feminist Studies* 13, 1987.

6. Helen King, *Hippocrates' Women: Reading the Female Body in Ancient Greece* (New York: Routledge, 1998), 28.

7. King 1998, 28–29; Miriam Yalom, *A History of the Breast* (New York: Ballantine Books, 1997), 206.

8. Plato, *Timeus* 91a-d; King 1998, 26.

9. See King 1998, 211.

10. King 1998, 213.

11. King 1998, 213.

12. Barbara Duden, *The Woman Beneath the Skin: A Doctor's Patients in Eighteenth-Century Germany*, trans. T. Dunlap (Cambridge: Harvard University Press, 1997).

13. Bordo (1995) has given a lovely reading of the threat of cravings and uncontrollable appetites in women (160–61).

14. See for example Lori B. Andrews, *The Clone Age: Adventures in the New World of Reproductive Technology* (New York: Holt, 1999); Donna J. Haraway, *Simians, Cyborgs and Women: The Reinvention of Nature* (New York: Routlege, 1991); Barbara Katz Rothman, *The Tentative Pregnancy: How Amniocentesis Changes the Experience of Motherhood* (New York: Norton, 1993); and Robbie Davis-Floyd and Joseph Dumit, eds., *Cyborg Babies: From Techno-Sex to Techno-Tots* (New York: Routledge, 1998).

15. Rüff, *De Conceptu et Generatione Hominus* (Francofurti ad Moenum: Christophorus Froscho, 1554, trans. London, 1637 as *The Expert Midwife*); Jacques Guillemeau, *Child-birth, or the Happy Delivery of Women* (London, 1635); François Mauriceau, *The Diseases of Women with Child and in Childbed* (Paris, 1694, trans. H.

Chamberlen, London: A. Bell, 1697); *The English Midwife Enlarged* (London: Rowland Reynolds, 1682); John Sadler, *The Sicke Woman's Private Looking-Glasse* (1636, reprinted London: Theatrum Orbis, 1977); Paul Portal, *The Complete Practice of Men and Women Midwives, or the True Manner of Assisting a Woman in Child-Bearing* (trans. London: H. Clark, 1705); Pierre Dionis, *A General Treatise on Midwifery* (trans. London: A. Bell, 1719); Nicholas Culpeper, *Directory for Midwives* (London: Peter Cole, 1656).

16. Harold Speert, *Obstetric and Gynecologic Milestones Illustrated* (New York: Parthenon Publishing Group, 1996), 191.

17. See Mirelle Laget, "Childbirth in the Seventeenth and Eighteenth Century France," in *Medicine and Society in France*, ed. R. Foster and O. Ranum (Baltimore: Johns Hopkins University Press, 1980).

18. See Karen Newman, *Fetal Positions: Individualism, Science, Visuality* (Palo Alto: Stanford University Press, 1996), especially 26–7.

19. Barbara Duden, *Disembodying Women: Perspectives on Pregnancy and the Unborn*, trans. L. Hoinacki (Cambridge: Harvard University Press, 1993), 43.

20. Although this purported audience of female patients cannot simply be taken at face value, given the very low levels of female literacy at the time, as Mary Fissell points out. See M. Fissel, "Hairy Women and Naked Truths: Gender and the Politics of Knowledge in *Aristotle's Masterpiece*," *The William and Mary Quarterly* 60:1, 2003, www.historycooperative.org/journals/wm/60.1/fissell.html.

21. For example, see Dionis 1719, 340, 342.

22. See especially *Aristotle's Masterpiece*, but each of these texts contains an extensive section on such monstrous births.

23. Guillaume Mauquest de la Motte, *A General Treatise of Midwifery* (trans. London: J. Waugh, 1746).

24. "When the Womb Went Bad: Motherhood in Sixteenth Century England," in *Vernacular Bodies: The Politics of Reproduction in Early Modern England* (New York: Cambridge University Press, 2004).

25. *Directory for Midwives* 1656.

26. *Child-Birth, or the Happy Delivery of Women*, trans. London 1635.

27. Dionis 1719.

28. *The Midwives Book, or the Whole Art of Midwifery Discovered* (1671, reprinted New York: Oxford University Press, 1999). This passage is in the context of a defense of the effectiveness of Hippocratic scent therapy as a means for cajoling the womb to move about within the body.

29. London, 1727.

30. *The Force of the Mother's Imagination upon her Foetus in Utero* (London: J. Walthoe, 1730).

31. Mauquest de la Motte 1746.

32. *Maternity Handbook for Pregnant Mothers and Expectant Fathers*, The Maternity Center Association of NYC (New York: Putnam and Sons, 1932), 14–15.

33. Sources for these and other examples can be found in Margrit Shildrick's *Embodying the Monster: Encounters with the Vulnerable Self* (Thousand Oaks: Sage Publications, 2002); this work also contains an excellent history and analysis of the maternal imagination. See also Sadler 1636, Turner 1730, and Culpeper 1651.

34. In fact, a picture of this case forms the frontispiece to *Aristotle's Masterpiece, or the Secret of Generation Displayed in All the Parts Thereof* (published anonymously in London in 1684), which is mostly devoted to alarmist tales of the ravages of maternal imagination upon the bodies of children.

35. Quoted in Turner. Interesting, this argument will be turned on its head a generation later, as we will see, when this same analogy between the bond of gestation and the bond of nursing will be used to argue that there is a direct transmission of properties from nurse to child through the milk and that nurse and child should in fact be seen as forming a unified entity. See chapter 2.

36. I discuss this transition in detail in chapter 3.

37. See Fissell 2004 for many, many examples of this.

38. See Shildrick 2002, 42ff., for an extended discussion of this point.

39. See Shildrick 2002 and sometimes Duden 1993 for this kind of one-sided feminist reading of the phenomenon.

40. See chapters 3, 4, and 7. See also Elizabeth Armstrong, *Conceiving Risk, Bearing Responsibility: Fetal Alcohol Syndrome and the Diagnosis of Moral Disorder* (Baltimore: Johns Hopkins University Press, 2003), for an excellent discussion of our interpretation of pregnancy outcomes as matters of individual maternal responsibility and as embodied expressions of maternal character.

41. Again, see Fissell 2004 for detailed evidence of this.

42. London: Edward Thomas, 1671.

43. See Mullin 2005; Susan Feldman, "From Occupied Bodies to Pregnant Persons," in *Autonomy and Community: Readings in Contemporary Kantian Social Philosophy*, ed. J. Kneller and S. Axinn (Albany: SUNY Press, 1998); and Naomi Wolf, *Misconceptions: Truth, Lies and the Unexpected on the Journey to Motherhood* (New York: Doubleday Books, 2001), for just a few examples out of many.

44. See for example Annie Oakley, *The Captured Womb: A History of the Medical Care of Pregnant Women* (London: Blackwell, 1984).

45. Duden 1997.1

46. In England, the rate at the time was around 12%; see www.plimoth.org/learn/history/myth/Deadat40.asp.

47. See chapters 4 and 7.

48. Armstrong 2003, 194.

49. *Essay on the Force of the Imagination in Pregnant Women* (London, trans. 1772).

50. For example, see the report recently published by President George W. Bush's Council on Bioethics, *Beyond Therapy: Biotechnology and the Pursuit of Happiness* (Washington, 2003).

2

Imbibing the Love
of the Fatherland

In this chapter I partially and temporarily shift my attention away from medical discourses and representations of maternal bodies and onto the place of these bodies in the modern philosophical, political, and aesthetic imagination. I also move forward chronologically, in both history and in the reproductive cycle, changing my focus from seventeenth-century obstetrics to the place of the lactating new mother in pre-Revolutionary and Revolutionary France. In particular, I here explore in detail the (surprisingly dramatic) place that Rousseau assigned to maternal bodies in his philosophical accounts of human nature and civic life and how Rousseau's thought (surprisingly dramatically) shaped the political and imaginative role of such bodies in Revolutionary ideology, imagery, and social reforms. In the next chapter I will bring the themes from my first two chapters together and look at how medical representations of maternal bodies transformed along with and in light of the shifts in civic and imaginative status that the maternal body underwent during the late eighteenth century.

Several writers have acknowledged Rousseau's definitive role in permanently changing the social significance of the maternal body, and especially the lactating body, as well as the pivotal role that Rousseau's imagination of the maternal body played in shaping Revolutionary imagery, policy, and ideology. And they have likewise agreed that these shifts permanently and deeply changed our broad social understanding of the responsibilities and the character of maternal bodies.[1] Rousseau transformed the project of forming human nature into a civic project appropriately monitored by public institutions, rather than just a private process governed by the logic of maternal excesses and restraint. Yet few have examined the conceptual and ideological conditions that would make sense of this enormous influence or seriously considered the philosophical context and details of Rousseau's thoughts on the subject. Here, I argue that Rousseau's use of maternal bodies ought to be understood as an outgrowth of central tensions in Enlightenment culture and thought and its accompanying picture of the relationship between human freedom and the claims of nature. Further, I claim that it is only against this background that we can really understand the power of Rousseauian images of maternality for the Revolutionary rethinking of the nature of the democratic state and its citizens.

"BEGIN WITH MOTHERS"

Although he wrote just a handful of comments on the topic, it is hard to overestimate the critical role that Rousseau assigned to the nursing mother in the founding of the just Republic and equally hard to overestimate the astonishing influence that these few comments had on the ideology and imagination of Revolutionary and Republican French culture. In his only extended passage on the topic of nursing, Rousseau writes in *Emile*,

> Do you want to bring everyone back to his first duties? Begin with mothers. You will be surprised by the changes you will produce. Everything follows successively from this first depravity [namely wet-nursing]. The *whole moral order* degenerates; *naturalness* is extinguished in all hearts; the touching *spectacle* of a family aborning no longer attaches husbands, no longer imposes respect on outsiders. . . . There are no longer fathers, mothers, children, brothers or sisters. They hardly know each other. How could they love each other? But let mothers deign to nurse their children, morals will *reform themselves*, nature's sentiments will be awakened in every heart, the state will be *repopulated*. This *first* point, *this alone*, will bring everyone *back* together. . . . From the correction of this simple abuse would soon result a general reform; nature would soon have *reclaimed* all its rights. Let women once again *become mothers*, men will soon become husbands and fathers again.[2]

The other 500 or so pages of *Emile* do not concern nursing, and indeed, maternal bodies make a quick exit altogether from the text after early in Book I, when Rousseau, in the character of the tutor, takes over Emile's upbringing and education. Yet this comment on the power and importance of the nursing maternal body was taken to be sufficiently central to the message of the work as to form the topic for its frontispiece by the time it was reprinted during the 1780s, on the brink of the Revolution. The frontispiece image shows a gaggle of women breastfeeding at the feet of a towering bust of Rousseau, with the caption "L'Education de l'Homme commence à sa naissance," or "The education of man begins at birth."

It will take time for me to unpack the many ways in which this passage transforms the social and imaginative place of the maternal body, but for now I just want to call attention to a few of its most striking features. Rousseau places mothers at the 'beginning' and the 'first point' in the moral remaking and transformation of the state and its citizens—indeed, mothers' nursing practices 'alone' will play this founding role. Furthermore, the *whole* moral order stands or falls on whether or not mothers nurse their children. Their doing so is associated twice with the *naturalness* of the sentiments of the children they nurse, and by extension of every citizen who shares a social order with these children. It is not just the actual act of nursing but the *spectacle* of doing so that is supposed to play such a crucial role in producing properly ordered souls, families, and states. By breastfeeding, women will 'become mothers,' and hence the nursing maternal body is equated with the maternal body *tout court*. And notice two particularly odd claims the passage makes. First, if mothers nurse their children and make a proper spectacle of doing so, then morals will *reform themselves, all on their own*, free of any agency. Second, the body of the nursing mother is supposed to effect a kind of *return*—the state will be 'repopulated,' nature will 'reclaim all of its rights,' and everyone will be 'brought back together.' The proper order that flows from the nursing maternal body is associated not only with a *natural* order but with a *nostalgic* order of nature from which we have presumably strayed.

The *moral* power granted here to the maternal body is striking, as is the social and civic centrality of this power. How in the world did Rousseau intend the mere performance of the act of nursing one's child to accomplish, automatically, this wholesale rewriting and remaking of the familial, moral, and civic orders? As we saw, the idea that the maternal body has the power to produce order and disorder is not new, but now this order and disorder have been expanded well beyond the boundaries of the fetal body, to society and indeed morality writ large. I pointed out in the previous chapter that in seventeenth-century medical texts, the maternal body was remarkably free of any imaginative significance beyond itself; civic language makes no appearance in any of these early discussions of the proper 'government' of the maternal body, and while a mother's morals were put to the test by the health of her infant, this too was portrayed as a private matter; there were no references to the place of the mother's body in any larger 'moral order.' None of the earlier discussions of how to keep the maternal body pure in order to guard against deformed babies laid any substantial ground for this dramatic picture of the magnitude of the maternal body's powers and responsibilities.

Furthermore, we immediately see that nature has taken on a new ontological and normative status in this passage, in comparison with the earlier works. Whereas before, the proper natural order was simply the order that nature would have as long as it remained pure and un-interrupted or uncorrupted by human intervention, here the proper natural order is something that needs to be *actively* restored through proper human practice. Our earlier writers sought to keep the womb pure by protecting the fetus from maternal influences, but Rousseau assigns mothers a positive role in producing properly ordered human and civic nature.

As it turned out, Rousseau's vision of the nursing maternal body and its critical responsibility for the civic and moral order played an astonishingly influential role in altering the social position, image, and meaning of the maternal body in France, as I will show in detail later in this chapter. George Sussman writes, "Rousseau's famous plea for maternal nursing in Book I of *Emile* . . . is the *locus classicus* of the eighteenth-century campaign against wet-nursing. Writers commenting a generation after the appearance of *Emile* on Rousseau's impact on infant care wondered at how the Genevan Philosophe had somehow succeeded in persuading mothers to nurse their children where so many physicians and moralists before him had failed."[3] Rousseau offered what turned out to be a touchstone picture of the role of the maternal body in an enlightened democracy, and as we will see, his new vision of the maternal body played a central iconographic and political role in the French Revolution, thereby setting the stage for the ideological life of the maternal body right up into present-day North America. There was nothing hermeneutically subtle about Rousseau's status as the prophet and patriarch of the French Revolution and Republic, and his views on motherhood and lactation clearly served as the hallmark of this status. To give just one example out of many, consider a 1794 drawing in which Rousseau is triply represented as the un-veiler of the 'truth' of the Revolution: Rousseau's head looms over an allegorical representation of the Republic, who is doing the unveiling, while the 'truth' unveiled is an androgynous naked figure with Rousseau's face and bared female breasts, seated next to a multi-breasted fertility statue, with her hand on the Social Contract and a copy of *Emile* at her feet (see figure 2.1)

Sussman and other scholars have remained surprisingly uncurious, it seems to me, as to how a single author could have had such a huge

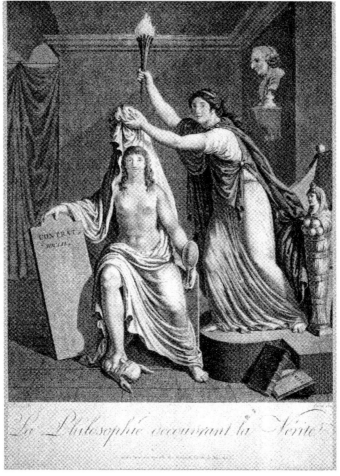

Figure 2.1. Jean Baptiste Gautier, after Boiseau, *Philosophy Uncovering Truth*, 1794, courtesy of the Museé Carnavalet, Paris.

influence. As Sussman points out, Rousseau's particular practical recommendations for child rearing and maternal nursing were foreshadowed by several authors, including in particular William Cadogan in his 1748 work *Essay upon Nursing and the Management of Children*, to which I will return later. Yet these earlier writings didn't cause much of a stir at the time, so Rousseau's extraordinary influence and visibility has to be explained in terms of some special readiness or need that existed in his *zeitgeist*. Poised on the brink of a revolution, late-eighteenth-century France was somehow ready to pragmatically and imaginatively adopt Rousseau's specific vision and to embrace and totemize Rousseau as a specific personality. In order to properly understand both Rousseau's transformation of the maternal body and the enormous impact and appeal of this transformation, we need to step back and situate Rousseau within his intellectual and political climate.

NATURE, CONTINGENCY, AND FREEDOM

The European Enlightenment of the seventeenth and eighteenth centuries, and its attendant humanism that became the conceptual and political bedrock of the French and American Revolutionary visions of the republican state, involved a radical rethinking of the fundamental relationship between human individuals, nature, and social and moral norms. One of the distinctive features of this historical movement—and one of the features that makes it such appealing territory for philosophers and intellectual historians—is that the tensions and developments within abstract philosophical discourse and within political practice were directly and explicitly intertwined. Revolutionaries read works of philosophy and used them to change the nature of the state, and philosophers used changing social institutions as direct fodder for metaphysical and ethical speculation. As Hegel would point out a generation later,[4] Rousseau was a paradigmatic example of a philosopher whose thought was constituted by that of his intellectual predecessors and constitutive of that of his political successors.

One of the central moves of the Enlightenment was the reduction of nature to a mechanical array, intrinsically devoid of norms and values and fully nomologically exhaustible, in contradistinction from the ancient, roughly Aristotelian picture of nature that had animated Western thought for two millennia. Along with this new picture of nature—a nature whose order could be mastered and predicted by science—came a movement of the seat of value to the individual agent. Neither an expression of God's will nor an inherent location of goals and purposes, Enlightenment nature became a playground for values imposed by humans rather than the source of these values. In turn, the individual who forged a system of values via his (sic) autonomous purposes and preferences formed the new, liberated lynchpin of normativity. On this humanistic picture, *self*-legislation becomes the criterion for the legitimacy of normative claims; cut free from the nomological reign of the natural and the divine, and enshrined as the source rather than the mere subject of normative claims, the individual becomes a being who is legitimately bound only insofar as he binds himself, through an exercise of his own autonomous will. The free, self-legislating individual—that cornerstone character of the Enlightenment—could not achieve this self-legislating status except by way of a denunciation of the legislative powers of God and nature. This self-legislating individual was at once the *product* of the draining of value from nature—for where else will value now be found?—and, equiprimordially, an ideal that *motivated* the attempt to read nature as brutely causal and non-normative. In turn, the protection and promotion of such self-legislating individuals became the humanistic goal of Enlightenment democracy.

Within this classic Enlightenment frame, however, *social* norms—the norms that bind us in virtue of our participation in a larger group—became deeply problematic. If self-governance is the hallmark of legitimate governance and the individual is the seat of legitimacy and value, then it is difficult to see how subjection to norms imposed by other humans could possibly count as anything other than heteronymous coercion. The problem seems to remain regardless of how these norms are selected, whether this is by majority vote, a constitutional legislator, or any other means. For how can we hope for more than a coincidental harmony of individuals' autonomously chosen principles, given that we can no longer infer an appropriate set of principles for governing individuals from nature itself? And if individuals' autonomously chosen principles differ, then any reasonably substantive set of social principles that governs them all will impose itself heteronymously on some. Emily Martin points out that a central feature of the Enlightenment was the "loss of certainty that the social order could be grounded in the natural order."[5] The humanistic individual was a self-grounding agent whose social bonds needed to be justified, for he had no *natural* place ordained for him within society. Social laws, it seemed, could only be contingent conventions, and as such they could legitimately bind individuals only if those individuals contingently chose the same principles for themselves. But this, of course, provided no grounding for a stable, unified, cooperative state with shared and legitimate laws. This dilemma—how can a law justly bind *me*, no matter how salutary its pragmatic effects, if I did not choose it myself?—is a familiar one. My point at the moment is not to articulate a new or contentious dilemma but to point out how this very familiar dilemma is not a timeless one, but rather one born out of the displacement of norms from nature to individuals, so characteristic of the movement of the Enlightenment.

The purest articulator of this dilemma may well also be the purest representative of Enlightenment ideology, namely the Marquis de Sade. Sade wrote during the peak of the Revolution, and soon afterward, Hegel would argue that Sade's vision was the inevitable—and self-destructive—conclusion of Enlightenment thought.⁶ In *Philosophie dans le Boudoir* and his other philosophical, pornographic parables, the Marquis argues that a true enlightened republic cannot fetter the rights of the individual in any way whatsoever, including the right to use or damage the body of another if it suits one's fancy. In the Marquis' potent vision, we cannot make the slightest sense of a human desire that is at odds with nature, for humans *are* natural beings. Our natures must therefore be directly identified with our selves, including our desires, and cannot be used as some sort of independent measure of the propriety of those desires. Any attempt to set up a normative tribunal over and above the immediate concreteness of human impulse is, in his view, a (covert if not explicit) attempt to smuggle God back into either nature or the state—and, as he puts it, the only appropriate reaction to this religious imposition is to throw shit upon its perpetrators in the public square.⁷ Of course, this vision can only support a nonstate—a state without laws and without any ability to coordinate social cooperation—which was just what the Marquis had in mind. His 'state,' such as it is, exists only to demand of its citizens that they self-legislate.⁸

But of course, most Enlightenment intellectuals were far from satisfied with Sade's social nihilism, even if it was arguably the fullest expression of their own metaphysical vision. For most of the humanist political theorists of the Enlightenment, the central question was how to avoid the Marquis' conclusion given his broad premises: that is, how could a group of free individuals with contingent preferences and wills come together into a stable whole unified by common laws? How could we design a republic that would be legitimate, where legitimacy had to be grounded in the autonomous self-legislations of individuals, and at the same time harmonious and cooperative? Or, as Rousseau put it in the most famous formulation of the problem, in *On the Social Contract*, how could we "find a form of association which defends and protects with all the common forces the person and goods of each associate, and by means of which each one, while uniting with all, nevertheless obeys only himself and remains as free as before?"⁹

I think that Rousseau is right that this is *the* fundamental political question for Enlightenment humanists, and he is also right to frame it in a way that brings out the Sadean near-paradoxicality of even searching for a solution. How can individuals unite with all and yet obey only themselves? I think that Rousseau's solution, furthermore, is in its barest essence the only possible solution: individuals must somehow come to jointly participate in a 'general will,' which is the will of all *and* the will of each, so that there can be no conflict between these two sources of legislation. Freedom can exist together with social unity only if subjection to the social principles cementing this unity is in fact voluntary self-subjection on everyone's part—a self-subjection that expresses rather than thwarts individual will. But of course, this just displaces and sharpens the central question, which is now this: Given that we are contingent beings with different wills and preferences, how can we possibly create or guarantee the existence of a shared general will that can be a legitimate source of normative claims? Once we remove God and nature as sources of true, authentic or proper value, how can we do more than *hope* that our separate and contingent ends will harmonize? On the other hand, if human freedom within society can at best be a coincidence, then what hope is there for the Enlightenment dream of the humanistic republic of autonomous citizens?

The late eighteenth century provided two basic responses to this dilemma, in addition to Sade's deflationary response, which we can call the 'rationalist' and the 'sentimentalist' solutions. The rationalist solution—crystallized in Kant—is to combine the thought that the *individual* must be the source of legitimate principles with the quest for a ground for *shared* principles, by arguing that a proper set of norms can be found, not in nature, but in rationality itself, as possessed by every autonomous individual. Reason itself dictates a set of universally valid principles to which we ought to freely subject ourselves. Though these principles are not 'up to us,' their claim on us is legitimate because true autonomy involves self-governance by reason rather than by the mute, contingent passions. We can be governed by common laws and yet obey only ourselves as long as we identify ourselves with our faculty of reason, abstracting from the bodily and passionate caprices that threaten to make up our empirical wills. Kant would make this solution famous just a few years after Rousseau's writings shaped the French Revolution, and it depends, for its success, upon a much-contested faith in the existence of universally valid rational principles substantial enough to lay the foundation for a humanistic, Enlightenment republic.

In contrast, Rousseau and most of his compatriots (including, prominently, David Hume and the Encyclopedists such as Diderot and d'Alembert) were sentimentalists and materialists who portrayed the human citizen as an essentially passionate, needy, contingent being whose identity was fundamentally mundane, and the human nation as a concretely located, contingent entity whose possible laws and forms of life were necessarily bound and shaped by time and place. For these authors, the human will was deeply seated in the concretia of the particular human body with its particular passions. Such a picture cannot reasonably look to a transcendent body of rational principles to solve the problem of uniting particular agents while keeping them free. Even if they believed that such a set of rationally binding principles existed, they would not think that we could simply identify our free wills with these principles. As passionate, needy beings routed in particular environments, our wills were, for these authors, much more mundanely determined and not simply intellectually redirectable. Furthermore, because the state was a located, contingent entity, the principles appropriate to it would have more content and more contingency than anything that would show up in something like formal Kantian moral law. A free *Frenchman* had to be not just a free *man* but a free *French* citizen, committed to participation in *that particular* republic, and with a particularized set of sentiments and needs that would let him be free within *that particular* social and material environment. (As Marx, continuing the sentimentalist tradition, would soon claim, the French need wine while the Germans need beer.) Rousseau spends the introduction of his *Discourse on the Origins of Inequality* spelling out the contingent, material conditions that he takes to be conducive to the possibility of a free and unified state, and he makes clear in this work and others such as *On the Social Contract* and *On the Government of Poland* that a legislator will have to tailor the laws of a republic to the specific contingencies of climate, national temperament, size, etc., that characterize his particular state.[10] Thus, as Terry Eagleton has argued at length, for the Enlightenment sentimentalists, the unity of free individuals in a Republican state needed to somehow be grounded in and arise out of a harmony among contingently determined mundane wills.[11]

This materialist, sentimentalist strand of the Enlightenment was what dominated public and political thought in pre-Revolutionary France, and it is in the context of this defining set of tensions surrounding individual freedom, Republican unity, nature, and law that we need to situate Rousseau's positive, constructive writings. In the face of the humanistic picture situating normative legitimacy in the contingent human individual, Rousseau needed to find a way of bringing citizens together under common laws without imposing upon their autonomous wills, in all of their contingency and their routedness in empirical nature.

This could only be possible, Rousseau reasoned, if individuals' contingent, mundane natures were of the *right sort* to lead them to choose these common principles out of their own free will. People's wills had to harmonize 'naturally' if they were to come together freely. However, old-fashioned found nature could no longer serve as any source of 'natural law' that would guarantee this unity—after all, one of the great Enlightenment advances was to free the individual from enslavement to mere found nature. Norms that are human products cannot be grounded in nature as it is on its own, and Rousseau has harsh words for those who try to legitimize human laws in some sort of given natural law.[12] Thus, Rousseau argued, our only option was to build legitimacy in the other direction, by *remaking* or *building* citizens' natures—we must inculcate in them the proper *second natures* so as to make them into beings who choose sociable principles and identify with the whole *of their own accord* and hence freely.

For Rousseau, the natural is a dynamic, shifting space, which we fashion even as we are fashioned by it. Asher Horowitz points out that in contrast to the Enlightenment conception of mechanistic nature defined in opposition to spirit or culture, Rousseauian nature is "historical and dialectical"; for Rousseau, there is no "abstract, static opposition between nature and artifice."[13] "We must not," Rousseau declares near the end of *Emile*, "confuse what is natural in the savage state with what is natural in the civil state."[14] Nature is mutable, indeed civilizable, and civilized nature can manifest and support human freedom rather than serve as its counterpoint. Indeed, Rousseau's writings are peppered with images of the cultivation, shaping, and taming of nature. When St.-Preux remarks upon the natural beauty of Julie's Elysium in Rousseau's novel *Julie, ou la Nouvelle Heloïse*, Julie responds, "It is true that nature made all this, but under my direction, and there is nothing here I did not arrange."[15] For Rousseau, then, nature is a realm that can be created and manipulated by us, rather than an immutable order to which we are passively subject. In the *Discourse on the Origins of Inequality*, we learn that human nature in particular is characterized by its *perfectibility* and that we are the agents of this process of self-transformation.[16] Perfectible nature is indefinitely improvable under the tutelage of the cultivating human hand.

When nature itself becomes a human product, then it can be invested with human principles and values from the ground up. On this vision, nature itself becomes the handmaiden of human freedom. Thus, in the guise of second nature, the natural comes to have normative force all over again. It is thus that Rousseau can open the *Discourse on the Origins of Inequality* with a quotation from Aristotle that in fact runs deeply against the grain of Enlightenment scientism: "Not in depraved things, but in those well oriented according to nature, are we to consider what is natural." Rousseau in effect finds a post-Enlightenment route to investing nature with human value, after its having been drained of it: nature will ground norms and serve as a source of legitimate principles, not by preempting the individual will but by being an expression of it.

This vision of nature turns the central task of the just legislator on its head. His main job is not to determine just laws and inscribe them in explicit legislation, but rather to foster appropriate second natures in citizens that will enable them to unify and yet choose according to their inclinations. He "must be capable of changing human nature, so to speak; of transforming each individual, who is by himself a perfect and solitary whole, into a part of a larger whole from which this individual receives, in a sense, his life and his being."[17] He must do this by intervening at the level of the mundane, molding people's habits, passions, inclinations and sentiments, building their natures from the ground up . . . for a central point here is that no mere *intellectual* indoctrination will do the trick. The most important sort of law, Rousseau says, is "not engraved in marble or bronze, but in the hearts of citizens. . . . I am speaking of mores, customs, and especially of opinion. . . . [The legislator] seems to confine himself to the particular regulations that are merely the arching of the vault, whereas mores, slower to arise, form in the end its immovable keystone."[18] The production of free, sociable citizens requires the molding of blind first nature into normatively infused second nature. The true *constitution* of the state is not its explicit laws but its natural constitution, in which the will of the citizens is grounded. Yet this natural constitution, like any constitution, must be designed by the legislator. True, legitimate natural law is a feat of human engineering.

Indeed, Rousseau claims that an individual nature, within civil society, cannot be left unshaped without condemning that individual to being a monster in fundamental conflict with his surroundings:

> Our species does not admit of being formed halfway. In the present state of things a man abandoned to himself in the midst of other men from birth would be the most disfigured of all. . . . Nature there would be like a shrub that chance had caused to be born in the middle of a path and that the passers-by soon cause to perish by bumping into it from all sides, and bending it in every direction.[19]

This vivid and moving passage is notable both for its explicit reliance upon the idea that nature is formed rather than given and its crucial notion that disfigurement is a context-dependent rather than an intrinsic feature of organisms. In civil society, first nature is in no way a normative touchstone of order; a citizen left to his first nature would in fact suffer *unnatural* disfigurement. The citizen needs to be designed so as to enable his possible well-ordered fit into the *new* 'natural order,' for otherwise this order will 'bump' into him rather than giving him a space to freely flourish. And, we can reasonably infer, a civil society that had no general program of human engineering, and was hence composed of a haphazard collection of 'misfits,' would not have *any* proper (second-) natural order into which citizens could fit and flourish without disfigurement. Hence the well-coordinated making of second nature is the critical condition for the possibility of an enlightened republic of free citizens. The true Republic will not merely coordinate individuals with distinct natures, it will *perfect* those natures themselves in order to make this coordination possible.

IMBIBING THE LOVE OF THE FATHERLAND

And now, finally, we have set the stage for the reintroduction of the maternal body. For how is this radical, orchestrated project of human engineering to be enacted? Clearly no one person could have the power that Rousseau officially assigns to the legislator—and indeed this legislator makes almost no appearances in Rousseau's writings outside of these few passages from *On the Social Contract*, which is remarkable given the enormity of the task he is assigned there. In practice, it is *mothers* to whom Rousseau assigns the responsibility for the making of second nature. Mothers—for better or for worse—mold new citizens at a level more fundamental and subterranean than that of their intellectual beliefs, commitments, and choices.[20] Abstract notions of the right are not sufficient, Rousseau believes, to actually shape the will, which gets its substantive content at the somatic level; our inclinations and sentiments are a matter of empirical nature, beginning with our first nature, as we come out of the womb, and shaped into our second nature as we are molded in childhood at the level of mundane practices, habits, and physical constitution. Prior to the age of reason, citizens have already been fundamentally molded at this somatic level by maternal forces. Mothers' bodies are responsible for the material production of our first natures, and once we are born, mothers' embodied care of infants and young children shapes the sentiments, habits, passions, and bodily constitution that make up second nature and that lay the ground for our exercises of will, reason, and social participation.[21] In this picture of the crucial political and ethical place of maternal caregiving, Rousseau closely follows Plato's discussion in Book IV of the *Republic* on the key role of the nurses, mothers, and early childhood practices in forming the bodily foundation for the properly free and civically appropriate citizen.[22]

This maternal shaping of nature is carried out, in the first instance, through the daily practices that make up early child rearing; it is a process determined by how mothers feed, dress, discipline, and speak to their children. But the maternal body serves as a powerful force governing human nature through a second mechanism: as a *spectacle*, the mother stands as a powerful symbol—*the* powerful symbol, for Rousseau—for the proper relationship between the state, or *patrie*, and its citizens. Just as the citizen must 'receive its life and its being' from the 'larger whole,' likewise the child at its mother's breast receives its nourishment from the larger whole of the maternal body. Properly presented, this spectacle is a key tool in inspiring appropriate *amour de la patrie* and the impulses and passions that constitute it.[23]

Now insofar as this bond between mother and nursing child appears as a 'natural' bond—one based on prediscursive, concrete unity rather than upon a civilized decision to associate—the spectacle of this bond can represent the Rousseauian ideal of a harmonious, well-ordered union of free citizens whose seamless participation in the general will is grounded in (second) nature, not in subjection to coercive or alien norms, nor in the happenstance of a mere contingent coincidence of ends. Thus the mother and child joined by milk become the symbol of the just Republic itself, which nourishes its citizens via a natural bond rather than protects them via a set of artificial conventions between separate individuals. At the same time this duo becomes an emblem of the proper site of the creation of this just Republic, namely maternal bodily practice and caregiving rather than the declaration of discursive principles. This elevation of the maternal body—and particularly the nursing maternal body—into a double-edged symbol and source of Republican health and harmony became one of Rousseau's most potent legacies, as we shall shortly see.

But in order for the nursing mother's body to do more than stand as a *symbol* for a set of social ideals—that is, in order for Rousseau to coherently impute to her actual nursing practices the pragmatic importance he gives them, the bond of milk must somehow be accorded a practical significance beyond that of nourishment. Indeed, Rousseau portrays mothers' milk as the *actual currency for the transmission of sociable second nature itself*. Citizens must come to love their countries *by nature*, so that this love is a spontaneous passion, and one written deeply into the makeup of the citizen body itself. This making of the passions from the inside out is accomplished by the ingestion of the right breast milk. In an absolutely crucial passage for my reading, Rousseau writes:

> It is education that you must count on to shape the souls of the citizens in a national pattern and so to direct their opinions, their likes and dislikes, that they shall be patriotic by inclination, passionately, of necessity. The newly-born infant, upon first opening his eyes, must gaze upon the fatherland, and until his dying day should behold noth-

ing else. *Your true republican is a man who imbibed the love of the fatherland, which is to say love of the laws and of liberty, with his mother's milk.* That love makes up his entire existence: he has eyes only for the fatherland, lives only for the fatherland; the moment he is alone, he is a mere cipher.[24]

I have italicized only a bit of this passage but nearly every word of it deserves emphasis. Much of the passage encapsulates neatly the elements of Rousseau's sentimentalist account that I have been exploring. Notice that it is by nursing that the infant imbibes *amour de la patrie*, and nursing involves having one's eyes upon the maternal body, while at the same time Rousseau starts by saying that the infant must begin by 'gazing upon the fatherland.' From all this we can infer that the maternal body *is*, in an important sense, a spectacle of the fatherland. This reading accords nicely with the rest of Rousseau's uses of maternal spectacle, and he finds rhetorical aid here from the serendipitous fact that *patrie*, which literally means fatherland, is actually a feminine noun in French. (See figure 2.2, in which *amour de la patrie*, or love of country, is explicitly represented as love of the mother, with her breasts available.) This passage also makes it explicit that mother's milk is a currency that transmits passions so that a proper maternal body/*patrie* will transmit proper love of that body with its milk.

The mother who nurses her own child thus becomes a patriot whose body is dedicated to carrying out her role in producing proper citizens, through the milk it offers and the spectacle of its own work that it provides. And her very patriotism transmits itself, through milk, directly to her child. As a result, 'morals reform themselves' without the need for any coercive or explicit interventions. Indeed, Rousseau portrays his contemporary social body as hysterically fractured, split open by divided loyalties, diversities in passions, and self-interested individualism (*amour proper*), all of which make any current unity under common social laws necessarily coercive rather than 'natural.'[25] The inarticulate bond of mothers' milk serves as an emblem, then, both for the cure for these fractures in the body politic and for its proper healed form. The maternal body becomes the critical origin, not only of the well-formed individual but also of the well-formed state and the possibility of human flourishing and sociability in general.[26]

Is this reference to 'imbibing the love of the fatherland' just a metaphor? In the previous chapter, we saw that the idea that passions and character could be transferred, very literally, from the body of the mother to that of her child was 'common knowledge' in the centuries leading up to Rousseau's writing—this knowledge was reported without a raised eyebrow in the most serious and respected medical works

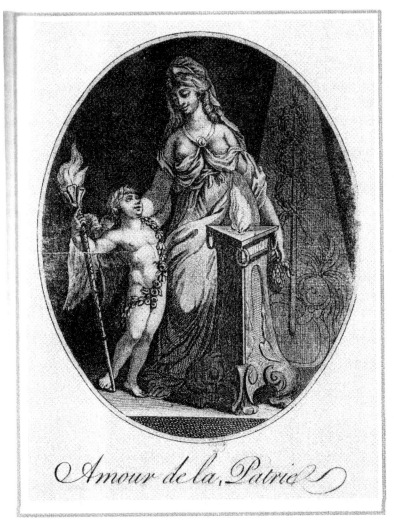

Figure 2.2. "Amour de la Patrie," 1793, courtesy of the **Bibliotèque Nationale.**

of the time. Whatever Rousseau's own beliefs were, there is no reason to think that at this time, readers would hear the reference to the transference of passions and character via breast milk as less than completely literal. In chapter 1, I looked at such transferences in the context of the purported effects of the maternal imagination during gestation; in the following section we will need to backtrack a bit in order to understand how breastfeeding, in particular, was understood by the medical community in the seventeenth and eighteenth centuries so as to situate Rousseau's comments in their proper context.

THE MEANING OF MILK IN THE SEVENTEENTH AND EIGHTEENTH CENTURIES

The importance and benefits of mothers nursing their own children, rather than sending them out to wet nurses, had been hotly debated in medical circles for quite a while by the time Rousseau came along. That the topic was one of passionate and frequent debate is clear from Culpeper's irreverent and impatient introduction to his own chapter on nursing: "Oh! What a racket do Authors make about this! What thwarting and contradicting, not of others only, but of themselves!"[27] Indeed, most seventeenth- and early-eighteenth-century obstetrical textbooks, including most of those we examined in the last chapter, contain at least a short discussion of the benefits of maternal nursing, as well as the principles for choosing a suitable wet nurse if the mother declines to nurse. Actually, one could almost say 'when' the mother declined to nurse, for it is clear from these writings both that maternal nursing was held as the medical and maternal ideal *and* that it was expected that almost all mothers would in fact make use of a wet nurse. Pierre Dionis is particularly explicit about this, writing in his preface, "This treatise concludes with an advice to mothers, to give suck to their own children, and though it is not expected that many will follow it, because they love their ease too much, and their children too little, yet we think ourselves obliged . . . to set before them the reasons."[28] In fact he devotes at least as much time to the principles for choosing a wet nurse as to the argument against wet-nursing. This structure is mimicked in many works of the time, which contain an argument for maternal nursing followed directly by rules for choosing wet nurses.[29] It is clear from these works that wet-nursing was the normal, accepted means of feeding infants at the time, even if ideologically it was seen as suboptimal.

The texts give elaborate directions for what wet nurses should eat and wear, how old they should be, what sort of 'constitution' they should have, and so forth. In each text, *nursing* refers most directly to feeding and lactation, but there is an unquestioned and pervasive assumption that the 'nurse' in this narrow sense will also be the primary caregiver. The chapters on nursing begin with lactation but move smoothly to discussions of how infants should sleep, what they should wear, how often they should go out, etc. Furthermore, they fold arguments about the importance of *raising* one's own children into their arguments for maternal lactation. In this metonymic identification of breastfeeding and caregiving—an identification that is firmly built into our ambiguous word *nursing* in its contemporary context—they certainly foreshadow Rousseau. This association may well have been substantially rooted in the realities of the social arrangements of the time, but it is important to notice how it underscores and gives imaginative grip to our image of milk as the incarnation of maternality, and it makes it difficult for readers to abstract the issue of feeding and suckling practices away from the larger significance of mothering, in the broader sense of nurturing and caregiving. I will return to this point at length in later chapters, but for now I just want to note that this tight association of suckling with caregiving as a whole certainly provided Rousseau with hospitable rhetorical soil in which to root the heavy responsibilities that he would assign to the nursing breast.

Reading backward from Rousseau, these seventeenth-century discussions of nursing are interesting with respect to what they do and what they don't contain. It is clear that just as the womb was seen as a literal medium of passions and character during gestation, the milk was seen as such a literal medium after birth: a great concern in all the discussions of choosing wet nurses is avoiding the transmission of the nurse's 'vices' through the milk. Culpeper refers (with humorous suspicion) to the many writers who insist that "the child draws his conditions from his nurse." Such a concern is continuous both with contemporaneous theories of the maternal imagination and with Rousseau's call for citizens who 'imbibe the love of the fatherland.'

However, despite these numerous discussions of the passing on of the vices of wet nurses, there are no early discussions of the possibility that *mothers* might pass on vices or virtues to their children through suckling.

That mothers might be at least as vice-ridden as the wet nurses they hired seems not to have registered as a possibility, perhaps because of assumptions about the social class of potential readers, and perhaps because the decision to nurse one's own child was deemed already sufficient evidence of an appropriately virtuous, maternal character. (We will see in the next chapter that this assumption certainly did not persist through the post-Rousseau era.) Some texts also make vague reference to a 'shared nature' between mother and infant that somehow is supposed to guarantee that the mother's milk is well suited to the infant and hence presumably not prone to corrupt that infant.

More interesting is the absence of any discussion of the potential of maternal breastfeeding for inculcating *virtues*, especially given Rousseau's heavy use of such vocabulary. I argued earlier that in the seventeenth century, nature was seen as an immovable benchmark;

the best that maternal practice could do, by way of shaping children's nature, was to refrain from interfering with it or distorting it. Nature could not be improved upon but only corrupted. It makes sense, in this context, that milk would not be seen as a tool for *enhancing* virtue. This difference should begin to suggest to us that the conception of nature itself underwent a significant shift between this era and Rousseau's, when breast milk becomes a primary tool for the perfecting of human nature.

Given that maternal bodies were not yet seen as capable of improving upon human nature, it makes sense that they would not be seen as significant sites of responsibility for shaping and reforming the body politic as a whole. And indeed, these early texts do not assign any of the ethical or civic significance to maternal nursing that we find in Rousseau. However, as we move through the eighteenth century and approach Rousseau's era, we can trace a shift in the medical dialogue surrounding nursing. In particular, two British works that were nearly contemporaneous with *Emile* are telling: Charles White's *A Treatise on the Management of Pregnant and Lying-In Women*[30] and William Cadogan's *Essay upon Nursing and the Management of Children from Birth to Three Years of Age*.[31] Both works still remain free of the political and ethical rhetoric that permeates Rousseau's writings, but they introduce a new element that is not present in the earlier works: They both make heavy use of a normative notion of 'following nature' in raising and caring for infants, and both argue for the importance of maternal breastfeeding by way of its 'naturalness,' in contrast to various 'unnatural' child-rearing practices.

White claims that maternal breastfeeding is what happens in the 'state of nature' and suggests that therefore wet-nursing is 'unnatural,' in the sense of being corrupt and deviant rather than merely artificial. In Cadogan's text, 'Nature' becomes a major structuring concept, one charged with fundamental normative weight and rights. Cadogan associates the natural *both* with science and its recent liberating and enlightening progress *and* with the proper, the appropriate, and the uncorrupted, so that intervening on the natural order becomes unscientific, perverse, and corrupt— "As if Nature, exact Nature, had produced her chief Work, a human creature, so carelessly unfinished as to want those idle Aides to make it perfect."[32] For after all, "The Art of Physick has been much improved within this last century; by observing and following Nature more closely, many useful Discoveries have been made, which help us to account for things in a Natural way."[33]

Following nature thus now becomes a principle for proper conduct and sound medical practice, in a way that was at least not rhetorically vivid in the earlier texts. These texts, we saw, treated uncorrupted nature as a pure benchmark toward which the management of the body should *aim*, but the route to protecting the natural was not particularly to 'follow' nature but to proactively manage it. There is a crucial difference between taking the natural—that excruciatingly and unendingly ambiguous and multivalent concept—as an *end* to protect and promote, as earlier writers did, and as a *guiding principle* that should shape and measure practices, as Cadogan does. Like Rousseau, Cadogan uses this principle of 'following nature' to justify recommendations such as not swaddling and making sure infants get lots of fresh air. And when he turns to breastfeeding, he writes: "Let us consider what Nature directs in this case: If we follow Nature, instead of leading or driving it, we cannot err. In the Business of nursing, as well as Physick, Art is ever destructive, if it does not copy this Original."[34]

In associating the natural with the 'original' and letting it serve as a source of normative direction, Cadogan here makes a Rousseauian move without precedent in the textbooks we looked at earlier. And yet, compared with Rousseau, Cadogan aligns himself much more closely with the traditional Enlightenment conception of nature. His nature is first and foremost the subject and object of science, so that science becomes the tool for regulating the maternal body. For Rousseau, we saw, nature serves as *both* a guide *and* a malleable medium that can be enhanced or perverted by human hands, while for the much more scientistic Cadogan, nature is still an absolute benchmark containing the fixed standards for proper practice within itself. At the same time, Rousseau, in a Romantic voice, emphasizes the intuitive and commonsense accessibility of 'natural' practices and the inherent knowledge possessed by maternal bodies when they are not corrupted by culture and reason. Cadogan, on the other hand, emphasizes the need for proper (masculine) scientific method to take over from the unsystematic meanderings of (maternal) intuition: "[The] Method of Nursing has too long been fatally left to the Management of Women, who cannot be supposed to have proper knowledge to fit them for such a Task, notwithstanding they look upon it as their own Province. What I mean, is a Philosophic Knowledge of Nature, to be acquir'd only by learned Observation and Experience, and which therefore the Unlearned must be incapable of."[35] Given this distrust of feminine, untutored intuition, it is no surprise that Cadogan asserts that he "would earnestly recommend it to every father to have his Child nursed under his own Eye, to make use of his reason and sense in superintending and directing the management of it."[36]

In enlisting fathers in the surveillance of the maternal body, Cadogan moves a crucial step closer to placing this body into a domain of social concern. In fact, Cadogan's text was commissioned by the governor of a foundling hospital (even though Cadogan generally presumes, in the text, that he is dealing with a traditional family unit). Such an assignment indicates that by this time, breastfeeding practices had become a matter of institutional and systematic social concern; Cadogan's text, though a medical text, was designed as part of a state apparatus providing social services. This too moves the maternal body into the public domain of surveillance and accountability in a way not seen in the earlier texts, which, as I noted, were explicitly designed to intimate works read by patients—in Sadler's words, to provide a "Private Looking-Glasse" for female patients.

Cadogan (and those he worked for) began to place the maternal body within the larger space of social institutions and to subject it to some social surveillance. This crucially prefigures (and perhaps helped to enable) Rousseau's elevation of this body into a social symbol and a privileged object for social surveillance. But Cadogan's lactating body, like his conception of nature, is transitional and not yet Rousseauian. Cadogan places the maternal body to some degree *under the control of* the social gaze, but this control is unidirectional. For Rousseau, this relationship will be bidirectional, for as we saw, the Rousseauian maternal body *exerts control through* being a spectacle and through nurturing and the inculcation of habits and passions. The spectacular power of lactation to heal and create proper social bonds—to *perfect* rather than just *preserve* nature—makes no appearance in Cadogan or earlier texts. When nature serves as a fixed benchmark, the social power of the lactating body—for both good and ill—is curtailed: the best it can do is follow nature and *fail to corrupt* the bodies and character of infants. It is not surprising, therefore, that Cadogan still does not invest either his text or the maternal practices he discusses with anything like the civic and moral meaning, promise, and responsibility that Rousseau does.

The idea that milk can serve as a concrete medium for transmitting character and sentiment is in fact an ancient one, dating back at least to the myth of Romulus and Remus. But what we have seen in this section is a transition under way in the status of the lactating body, occurring in the midst of renegotiations of our notions of nature, maternality, and spectacle. Cadogan discloses a moment when breastfeeding bodies were on their way from being private matters to public and institutional objects of concern and spectacle, and the natural was on its way from being a fixed benchmark that could be corrupted or preserved to a source and subject of normative principles of order, harmony, and virtue. In the earlier texts, treatments and interventions into the maternal body were not themselves unnatural, for unnaturalness was a matter of internal deformity, to be prevented by whatever means. By Cadogan's time, nature had gone from a *form* to a *principle*, from a static touchstone to a measure of dynamic practices.

LITERAL AND FIGURATIVE LACTATING BODIES

Before our detour through medicine, I asked the following question: Did Rousseau believe that it was literally maternal breast milk *itself* that was so critical for the proper physical, moral, and sentimental development of infant-citizens—that is, for the production of proper second nature? We have found historical and medical precedents that show that the idea that sentiment and character could be literally transmitted through milk—that infants could actually 'imbibe the love of the fatherland'—would not have seemed far-fetched at the time. On the other hand, it might be that Rousseau just believed that the lactating maternal body performed its social and moral work through its role as symbol and spectacle. His own texts are equivocal and underdetermining. Often his emphasis is on the role that the *image* of the nursing mother plays in stimulating proper sentiments among fathers, infants, and citizens. Certainly he does not see fit to offer any mechanistic story about how milk would transmit passions and virtues. On the other hand, his vitriolic attack on wet nurses seems literal and sincere enough.

Indeed, there was certainly good reason, from a public health perspective, to decry the concrete practice of wet-nursing at the time, given the rates of illness and mortality among wet-nursed babies.[37] Furthermore, Rousseau's own mother died in childbirth, and he was raised, sickly and weak, on the milk of a wet nurse. By his own reports he ended up not just physically compromised, but a 'monster' whose nature was deformed in such a way as to render him incapable of finding a harmonious place within society that would let him be free.[38] He was an exile from his country of birth and from regions of his country of residence—a country in which he resided tenuously as an expatriate and a sharp critic. By no standards did he count as a patriot harmonizing by nature with his fellow citizens.

Either way, the citizens of Revolutionary France drew nothing like a fine distinction between the nursing mother as a figurative symbol and as a literal source for Republican identity, and so in some sense the question of Rousseau's understanding of his own project is historically moot. Post-Revolutionary Republican France uncritically adopted the Rousseauian idea that the nursing mother was the proper mother of the Republic itself and that nursing was the medium of mothering.

Many of the uses of the maternal breast in Republican rhetoric and policy drew no neat distinction between this breast as concrete medium, as symbol, and as spectacular source of Republican values and identity. In 1791, the female citizens of Clermont-Ferrand wrote a letter to the French National Assembly, in which they boasted, "We see to it that our children drink an uncorrupted milk and we clarify it for that purpose with the natural and agreeable spirit of liberty."[39] Republican intellectuals dreamed up fictions of 'natural' republics in which women were formally honored for each child they breastfed. The French National Convention legislated that in national festivals, nursing mothers would receive public pride of place behind only public officials.[40] Patricia Ivinski writes, "After the Revolution, Rousseau's advocacy of maternal breastfeeding entered the public realm of political discourse under the new Republican government. In the decade following the events of 1789, Republican ideology promoted mother's milk as being capable of transmitting moral as well as patriotic virtues to children, the future of the Republic; articles in the popular press reminded mothers that their children 'must imbibe the principles of the Constitution from infancy,' both literally and figuratively linking maternal breast-feeding with Republican ideology."[41]

To a *limited* extent we can separate and identify three different, although mutually supportive and interdependent, civic appropriations of the maternal breast: the symbolic, the spectacular, and the literal:

1. In the wake of Rousseau, the French Republic routinely used nursing or bare-breasted women as symbols of the Republic, thereby picking up on the symbolic role that Rousseau assigned to the nursing body. Lactating women festooned Republican monuments, fountains, state-sponsored art, and other sites for public viewing. Indeed, the bare-breasted woman notoriously became the symbol of liberty herself, where liberty was incarnated in the well-ordered state composed of citizens nurtured into having proper natures; the preservation of liberty within society was the humanist dream that Rousseau's proposals were designed to promote.[42] By 1850, the bare-breasted woman representing France had been named Marianne and become an entrenched and familiar figure in European iconography.

2. These images of lactating Republican women were at one and the same time designed to *represent* the Republic—the 'mother' of the citizens—symbolically, and also to *mold Republican passions* through the spectacle of nurturance and unity they presented. The idea that art could stir up morally and politically proper passions was not new, of course, but

Rousseau had perpetrated a theory of human nature in which such passions actually *constituted identity*; hence the right images would play a foundational role in actually creating and sustaining the Republic, by creating and sustaining Republican citizens. Lactation imagery was used in a directly Rousseauian fashion by architects and supporters of the Revolution, to capture Republican ideals in aesthetic form, but also to promote them at the level of the passions. Both the male citizens and the mothers of these citizens were supposed to be not just appreciative of but *altered by* this imagery. Robespierre, David, and other masterminds of the Revolution staged several festivals to spectacularize and celebrate the nursing mothers of France in order to stimulate civic pride and identity.[43]

3. Meanwhile, Rousseau's dictum that Republican mothers should nurse their own babies and thereby transmit Republican values and identity could not have been taken more literally, and accordingly, the literal, concrete body of the nursing mother became highly politicized during the Revolution. The actual transmission of breast milk took on a purported civic significance that far outstripped its narrowly medical significance. Shortly before the Revolution, less than 5% of all Parisian babies were nursed by their mothers, and the overwhelming majority were sent out of the city altogether to live with rural wet nurses.[44] But in 1793, the president of the French National Convention officially declared that French mothers should breastfeed so that "military and generous virtues could flow, with maternal milk, into the hearts of all the nurslings of France."[45] That same year, the Convention decreed that only mothers who nursed their own children would be eligible for certain kinds of state support. With this decree, infant feeding practices and maternal bodies moved explicitly and dramatically into the sphere of civic regulation and responsibility. This legislation "signified governmental appropriation of the maternal breast as a political instrument."[46] The first move to institutionalize maternity leave in France began at this time as well.[47] This move helped transform mothering itself from a private practice to a state-sanctioned activity, with corresponding protections and civic responsibilities.[48] Art and public policy were both marshaled as complementary tools for encouraging the concrete practice of breastfeeding. One art critic, responding to a heavily exhibited painting of a baby preferring a wet nurse to his own

mother, commented, "May she [the mother] submit to the advice given in this painting, how many tears would she spare herself! It must be a cruel punishment for a mother to see her child, from the cradle, deny nature!"[49] By 1794, Prussia had jumped on the French ideological bandwagon, requiring all mothers to breastfeed by law.[50] By 1801, a full 51% of Parisian mothers nursed their children—up more than 1,000% in the course of twenty years. And although the institutionalized practice of wet-nursing continued, in curtailed but recognizable form, throughout the nineteenth and even the early twentieth centuries in both the old and the new world, the French bureau of wet nurses shut down permanently in 1876.[51]

Rousseau thus initiated a series of dramatic changes in the public status and concrete practices of maternal bodies, especially nursing bodies. He transformed nursing into the "first duty" of mothers, as the *Encyclopedia* of Diderot and his friends put it. Even Rousseau's critics, such as Mary Wollstonecraft, did not dare to call into question the Rousseauian tenet that nursing is a civic duty crucial to the production of sympathetic and well-ordered citizens. Rousseau changed the symbolic and imaginative value and function of the maternal body; sparked revisions in the standards and social arrangements governing mothering practices; brought together medical, aesthetic, and political discourses with respect to maternal bodies; and transformed these bodies from private, almost furtive matters into vivid centers of public management, surveillance, celebration, approbation, and regulation. In his wake, medical discourse surrounding maternal bodies would be deeply marked and shaped by moral and political language and concerns. The maternal body had become an essentially normatively charged medium, heavily burdened with civic hopes and responsibilities. Although I have argued that Rousseau's thought could take the shape and have the influence it did because of the historical and intellectual conditions present in Enlightenment France, and although I have tried to show that shifts and transformations in the understandings and practices of nature and maternality were already under way in Europe prior to Rousseau's writings, we still have to say that he brought about nothing short of a revolution in the configuration of the maternal body. And, I will argue in the second half of this book, this revolution has so far proved permanent; contemporary maternal bodies are imagined, represented, and treated within a fundamentally Rousseauian framework.

FIRST AND SECOND NATURE

But Rousseau's picture of the place of the maternal body in social space is actually more conflict-ridden and double-edged than these Republican appropriations of it make it seem. In order to understand why this is, we need to return to this shifting, trickster notion of nature itself and interrogate Rousseau's version of it more carefully. I have already argued that this notion was in flux in the seventeenth and eighteenth centuries, but Rousseau's version of it was more complicated and equivocal than that of his predecessors and foreign contemporaries.

I introduced Rousseau's appeal to 'natural' mothering as his means to solve the humanistic problem of nature's *in*ability to ground social norms, and we can go no further without acknowledging the tensions that this already introduces into the heart of Rousseauian nature. The image of the nursing mother as the source and symbol of 'natural' harmony and 'natural' practices is one that gets its rhetorical force through its associations with a naïve notion of originary, 'first' nature—of nature *as opposed* to culture, rather than nature as the handmaiden of culture. We saw Cadogan, for instance, using such a notion of nature as a normative concept. Rousseau's language of 'reclaiming,' 'reforming,' 'repopulating,' and 'reuniting' trades on the idea that human nature imbibed through the maternal breast is good in and through its ability to *return* us to a natural state prior to the degradations, deformations, and coercions of culture. Culture corrupts and disfigures, producing monsters, the lore goes, and likewise a 'return' to nature heals and restores order.

But the 'nature' in which Republican virtue is instilled, and through which the harmony of the social whole is cemented is, as we saw, not first but *second* nature. Indeed, we saw that Rousseau *began* from the insight that first nature could not provide *any* normative grounding for a social order, and that it was specifically contingent social sentiments such as the love of a particular country that were supposed to be inculcated by mothers in order to produce second-natural harmony and freedom. The maternal breast not only shapes nature by transmitting passions, but the passions it is supposed to transmit are ineliminably and specifically social, not just general fellow-feeling, for instance, but a love of *this particular* country, laws, and citizens. (See figure 2.3, where the Republican crest on a nursing baby's bonnet symbolizes this imbibing of a highly enculturated, socially specific identity.) The natures instilled at the maternal breast get their *normative* status as *proper* natures only when they succeed in *perfecting* first nature in accordance with the contingent needs of the state.

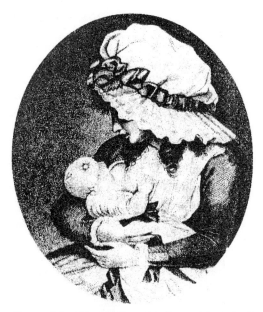

**Figure 2.3.   "Republican Mother with Child,"
1793, courtesy of the Bibliotèque Nationale.**

Julia Kristeva characterizes the maternal body as "a strange fold
that changes culture into nature . . . in order to pass on the social
norm."[52] We are used to thinking of human work as transforming nature into culture, but the Rousseauian/Revolutionary maternal body
has the opposite task. When culture leaves nature behind, it also
leaves behind the predictability, stability, and harmony of a fixed order. In order to bring stable harmony and order back into culture, the
responsibility for doing so is passed to mothers' bodies, which are
called upon to re-embed culture back into nature again. Nature becomes the vessel of culture, whose norms are 'passed on' through our
bodies. But this enculturated nature is not and never will be simply
the same as originary nature. If it were, it would not be responsive to
culturally contingent needs, nor would it properly embed cultural
norms and the general will. For all his rhetoric of return, Rousseau
must be seen as making use of a substantially more dynamic and his-
toricized notion of nature than his Enlightenment predecessors—one
in which nature cannot be assumed to be unmarked by or prior to culture, even as it serves as culture's ground.
     This new nature is vividly represented in a French print from 1794
entitled "La Nature," which represents nature as a white woman
suckling a child at each breast. Though the children are the same size

and apparently the same age, one is black and one is white (see figure 2.4). Here nature presumably stands for the 'natural' Republic—represented, once again, by a breastfeeding woman—offering its nurturance to all citizens regardless of differences. This is the standard commentary on the picture.[53] Indeed, the notion that the Republic, as a lactating woman, had a bosom that was open to all was itself a recurring theme in art and rhetoric.[54] This image plays off the idea that a just republic that nurtures and unifies its citizens is a natural republic, governed by natural order and unity. But of course, taken literally, the image of a woman breastfeeding children of the same age and dif-

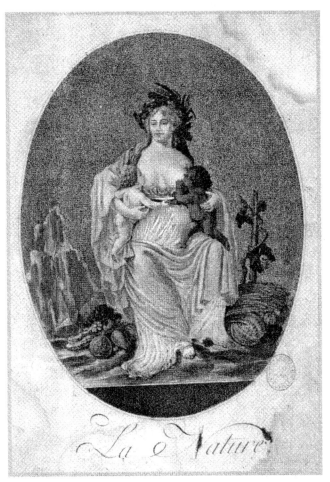

Figure 2.4.   Chez Basset, "La Nature," 1794, courtesy of the Museé Carnavalet, Paris.

ferent races is deeply 'unnatural' in the first-nature sense. How did she acquire these babies? Miscegenation was itself not seen as the most 'natural' reproductive arrangement at the time. But even if we assume that viewers could have accepted the black baby as this mother's natural child, it is impossible that both children could be, since they would have to have been gestated at the same time and have had different fathers. But perhaps these are not her biological children, in which case the image poses social rather than biological challenges to the viewer. However, if they are not her children, then she is presumably serving as their wet nurse, subverting the 'natural' bond of mother and child and serving as a strange icon of natural motherhood in the anti-wet-nursing climate of the post-Rousseauian Republic. Of course it is not hard to come up with plausible 'natural' explanations of the picture. But as an *image*, despite the flowery font and dripping plants evoking nature, its resonances, especially at the time, would have suggested a deeply *un*natural scene in the first-nature sense. The stark difference in races between the babies, and the image of a black child put to a white breast, surely would add up to a representation of a subversively unnatural maternal body. The picture sets up an ideologically charged image of a new kind of nature: enculturated nature, which establishes order, unity and harmony; bridges differences between citizens; subverts and levels traditional power differences based on blood; and provides nourishment. This is decidedly not a return to first nature.

Such imagery, together with Rousseau's rhetoric, helps establish a new understanding of morally and socially appropriate nature as second nature, inculcated by mothers. But, given that social harmony and human freedom depend on this contingent, corruptible process of inculcation, how shall we be sure that it is correctly executed? Unlike first nature, the nomological order of second nature is neither given nor fixed, but rather dependent upon the habits and practices of childhood and maintained through adulthood through ritual, festival, spectacle, and other subdiscursive mechanisms. And importantly so, for remember, second nature must bend itself to the contingent needs of different social contexts. Therefore mothers, as wielders of second nature, could inculcate the *wrong* natures, causing disorder, conflict, and general social disfigurement and monstrosity.

Rousseau's 'solution' is to draw upon images and metaphors of *first* nature as directives for mothers' practices. We ensure that mothers' bodies generate natural harmony and sociability rather than chaos by making sure that they follow 'nature' in their child-rearing practices. First and foremost is the directive to suckle their own children rather than create 'denatured nurslings' by introducing an 'unnatural' bond with a wet nurse who has no natural connection to the child.[55] He thus figures second nature as different from first nature and yet as trustworthy in virtue of its resonances with first nature. The association of second nature with the inarticulate, bodily bond of milk provides an image of order and unity. The physical bond of breast to mouth feels more substantial and perhaps trustworthy than a stipulated, 'artificial' union of separate beings via laws, covenants, or intellectual decisions.

But how can the appeal to a first-natural process such as maternal breastfeeding actually reassure us that this process will *properly* inculcate second nature? How is the purported (first) 'naturalness' of maternal breastfeeding supposed to ensure the (second) 'naturalness' of the unity and harmony of citizens, given the gap between these two senses of 'nature'? (Along the way, it's worth noting that communal breastfeeding and wet-nursing had been common practices throughout human history, while exclusive mothering was a rather new idea produced along with the modern bourgeoisie, so the sense in which nursing one's own child was supposed to be a first-nature practice is itself worth interrogating.) Upon reflection, the appeal to nature here seems dangerously circular: we use second nature to ground norms whose ground was lost when first nature was stripped of its normative character, and we trust the process by which second nature is instilled in virtue of its apparent naturalness in the first, precultural state. There is no tension in claiming that it is the first-nature practice of breastfeeding that serves as the mechanism transmitting second-nature sentiments and identities. However, we cannot consistently use the normative status of first nature as the guarantor of the normative propriety of instilled second nature at the same time as we claim that second nature has replaced first nature as the ground of legitimate social norms.

Ultimately, the Rousseauian connection between first and second nature is associative and imagistic rather than grounded in any coherent single understanding of the natural. Rousseau's thrusting of second nature to the forefront in discussions of human nature was a philosophically important advance over former rationalistic, voluntaristic, or mechanistic understandings of this nature emerging out of the Enlightenment. But he cannot consistently allow second nature to inherit the normative power of the first nature it has left behind. Nor is it at all clear that first nature itself retains any of this power in the wake of both humanism and Rousseau's dynamic, provisional understanding of nature in general. Despite the rhetorical weight of Rousseau's appeal to first nature in granting some practices the power to create proper second nature, there is no prima facie reason why we should actually believe that following first nature should particularly increase our chances of successfully inculcating proper second nature. Breast milk would seem to stand no greater chance of carrying the specific passions and virtues of French Republican identity when its source is the "natural" maternal body. Symbols of first nature may effectively *stand for* well-ordered second nature in imagination and representation, but this does not mean that we can turn this metaphor into a technique for producing this well-ordering.

The *imaginative* link that Rousseau forges between first nature and proper second nature was accepted without much interrogation or argument by Rousseau's Revolutionary followers. The Revolutionaries did not thematize the distinction between first and second nature—although as we just saw, some understanding of the distinction made its way into art. They plumped instead for a faith that 'natural' practices were the guarantors of well-ordered individuals—a faith that rests on an equivocation between these two natures and that flourishes still in the form of unargued commitments to the idea that 'natural' childbirth, child care, medications, etc., will somehow result in better 'natures' than their 'artificial' counterparts. Again, this turn is particularly ironic given that Rousseau's thought emerged out of the very humanism that *denied* first nature the capacity to ground norms and govern human practices. One of the only Revolutionary thinkers who worried explicitly about the paradoxes surrounding the dictum to follow nature in a humanistic age was the Marquis de Sade, who concluded that truly following the dictates of secularized, unenculturated first nature would lead not to sociability but to random and conflicting acts of unreasoned human caprice—and he was kept in jail for his troubles.

Rousseau himself, on the other hand, had quite a bit of ironic distance from his own rhetoric and was troubled by the necessary gap between first and second nature, and by the corresponding contingency involved in inculcating second nature. In particular, *given* that the principles of first nature that governed maternal bodies *underdetermined* the second-nature virtues and passions they were charged with inculcating, he worried that despite his own soothing rhetoric, the maternal body and breast could as easily corrupt, disfigure, and fracture the body politic through its citizen bodies as it could unite and perfect it. With the maternal power to enable freedom and sociability through inculcating proper form comes the corresponding power to deform and enslave, to produce monsters instead of virtuous patriot-citizens. Both the beginning of *Emile*, as we saw, and the *Lettre à M. d'Alembert* contain vivid descriptions of the dangers of the wayward maternal body that does not sustain the proper bond of milk or perform the proper spectacle of domesticity.

In Rousseau's hands, then, the maternal breast became not only the symbol of the possibility of social harmony and freedom but also the storehouse for anxieties over the contingency of this well-ordering. Despite pinning his hopes on it, Rousseau, like many others throughout history, profoundly distrusted the female body to do its job properly, seeing it as 'naturally' prone to temptation, corruption, and caprice. "A child spends six or seven years in the hands of women," he frets, "victim of their caprice and his own."[56] If women's first nature is morally and socially ambivalent, then it will ultimately serve as an ambivalent foundation for second nature as well.

We can throw Rousseau's double-edged relationship to the breast into vivid relief by contrasting his signal call to the maternal breast with which I began this chapter—a breast with the *natural* power to reform morals, build virtue, and establish order—with one of the most bizarre episodes in the *Confessions*:

> If there is one incident in my life which plainly reveals my character, it is the one I am now going to describe. . . . I entered a courtesan's room as if it were the sanctuary of love and beauty; in her person I felt I saw the divinity. . . . "This thing which is at my disposal," I said to myself, "is Nature's masterpiece and love's. Its mind, its body, every part is perfect. . . . Either my heart deceives me, deludes my senses and makes me the dupe of a worthless slut, or some secret flaw that I do not see destroys the value of her charms and makes her repulsive to those who should be quarrelling for possession of her." I began to seek for that flaw with a singular persistence. . . . Just as I was about to sink upon a breast which seemed about to suffer a man's lips and hand for the first time, I perceived that she had a malformed nipple. I beat my brow, looked harder, and made certain that this nipple did not match the other. Then I started wondering about the reason for this malformation. I was truck by the though that it resulted from some remarkable imperfection of Nature and, after turning this idea over in my head, I saw as clear as daylight that instead of the most charming creature I could possibly imagine I held in my arms some kind of monster, rejected by Nature."[57]

This tale of a monstrous female breast vividly reveals Rousseauian tensions that the Revolution would unwittingly inherit. It is *first* nature—nature 'about to suffer a man's . . . hand for the first time'— that is guilty of monstrosity and betrayal here. First nature is guilty of imperfection, even deformity, and—worse yet—there is no telling from all but the most intimate contact whether we are confronted with a trustworthy or a monstrous feminine body. But if first nature can thus betray us, then second nature that is built in its name is similarly untrustworthy. The natural breast may be Rousseau's best hope, but it cannot be counted upon either to embody order rather than monstrosity or to show its hand to the outsider's gaze.

NOTES

1. See Joan Landes, *Visualizing the Nation: Gender, Representation and Revolution in Eighteenth Century France* (Ithaca: Cornell University Press, 2001); George Sussman, *Selling Mothers' Milk: The Wet-Nursing Business in France* (Urbana: University of Illinois Press, 1982); Linda Zerilli, *Signifying Woman: Culture and Chaos in Rousseau, Burke, and Mill* (Ithaca: Cornell University Press, 1994); and Patricia R. Ivinski et al., *Farewell to the Wet-Nurse: Etienne Aubry and Images of Breast-Feeding in Eighteenth Century France* (Williamstown, MA: Sterling and Francine Clark Art Institute, 1998).

2. *Emile, or On Education*, trans. A. Bloom (New York: Basic Books 1979), 46, my emphasis.

3. Sussman 1982, 27.

4. See for instance Hegel's section on "Absolute Freedom and Terror" in the *Phenomenology of Spirit*, trans. A. V. Miller (New York: Oxford University Press, 1977).

5. Martin, *The Woman in the Body: A Cultural Analysis of Reproduction* (Boston: Beacon Press, 1987), 32.

6. Again, see Hegel's section on "Absolute Freedom and Terror" in the *Phenomenology of Spirit*.

7. From the pamphlet entitled "Yet Another Effort, Frenchmen, if You Would Become Republicans," embedded within his *Philosophie dans le Boudoir* (translated and reprinted in *Justine, Philosophy in the Bedroom, and Other Stories*, New York: Grove Press, 1990). In my view, Sade is most productively read as using this view as much to deconstruct Enlightenment ideology by pushing it to its limits as to promote it. However, his intentions do not matter here, as I am interested only in his purified humanistic picture of the individual as the seat of norms.

8. See Slavoj Zîzek's compelling reading of Sade in his "Kant and Sade: The Ideal Couple," at www.lacan.com/frameXIII2.htm.

9. *On the Social Contract*, trans. D. A. Cress (Indianapolis: Hackett, 1987), 24.

10. See Rousseau, *On the Social Contract*, as well as his *Discourse on the Origins of Inequality*, trans. Donald A. Cress (Indianapolis: Hackett Publishing Co., 1992), and *The Government of Poland*, trans. Willmore Kendall (Indianapolis: Hackett Publishing Co., 1985). See also Nicole Fermon's emphasizing of this dimension of Rousseau's thought in her *Domesticating Passions: Rousseau, Woman and the Nation* (Hanover, NH: Wesleyan University Press, 1997).

11. Terry Eagleton, *The Ideology of the Aesthetic* (New York: Blackwell, 1990).

12. *Discourse on the Origins of Inequality*, 13.

13. Asher Horowitz, *Rousseau, Nature and History* (Toronto: University of Toronto Press, 1987), 37, 50.

14. *Emile*, 406.

15. *Julie, ou la Nouvelle Heloïse* (Paris: Editions Garnier Frères, 1961), 254, my translation.

16. *Discourse on the Origins of Inequality*, 149.

17. *Social Contract*, 39.

18. *Social Contract*, 48.

19. *Emile*, 27.

20. For an extended discussion of mothers' role in the production of human nature and sociability that is more or less compatible with my own reading, see Fermon 1997.

21. See Book I of *Emile;* the preface to the *Discourse on the Origins of Inequality;* Rousseau's *Letter to d'Alembert* (reprinted in *Politics and the Arts,* trans. A. Bloom, Ithaca: Cornell University Press, 1968); and his posthumously published prequel to the *Social Contract,* the Geneva Manuscripts (reprinted in *The Collected Writings of Rousseau Volume 4,* trans. R. Masters and C. Kelly, Hanover, NH: University Press of New England, 1994).

22. And indeed, in Book I of the *Confessions,* Rousseau is explicit about the founding role of Plato's *Republic* in his thought. His *Discourse on the Origins of Inequality, Government of Poland,* and *Letter to d'Alembert,* among other writings, all cast his theory of civic association as a return to ancient principles. This contrasts with standard attempts to read Rousseau as a modernist for whom adherence to an abstract contract in the legacy of Hobbes and Locke is the foundation of the proper republic.

23. See for instance *Emile* (361, as well as the long passage from that work, which I quoted at the start of this chapter); Rousseau's *Discourse on the Origins of Inequality,* 9; and the *Letter to d'Alembert,* 129–36, where Rousseau recommends staging civic festivals in which dancing young women in modest dress be put on display in order to build public virtue through the spectacle they offer. Much of the *Letter* is devoted to the kinds of spectacles that women can create, as well as the power of these spectacles to form and to deform the bodies and characters of individuals and states. See also my "Performing Nature in the Letter to M. d'Alembert," in *Rousseau on Arts and Politics: Autour de la Lettre d'Alembert,* ed. M. Butler (Ottawa: Pensées Libres, 1998), 67–77.

24. Rousseau, *The Government of Poland,* 19.

25. See chapter 3 for a detailed discussion of this notion of the hysterical fracturing of the body politic.

26. In *A History of the Breast* (New York: Ballantine Books, 1997), Miriam Yalom argues that in the Netherlands in the seventeenth century, lactating mothers were already treated as seats of civic responsibility, as the secular Dutch republic invested the mundane, domestic domain with the spiritual significance formerly reserved for the divine (see her chapter 3). This predates the shift I am pinning on Rousseau. But as Yalom describes it, mothers there were seen as integral parts of a flourishing nation, but they were not called upon to stand for or be the originary condition for this nation itself. Hence their bodies were not politicized or marshaled as public symbols in the same way as they soon would be in France.

27. Nicholas Culpeper, *Directory for Midwives* (London: Peter Cole, 1656).

28. Pierre Dionis, *A General Treatise on Midwifery* (trans. London: A. Bell, 1719).

29. See in particular Guillaume Mauquest de la Motte, *A General Treatise of Midwifery* (trans. London: J. Waugh, 1746), as well as Culpeper 1656.

30. London, 1773, reprinted by Canton, MA: Science History Publications, 1987.

31. London, J. Roberts, 1748, reprinted in M. and J. Rendle-Short, *The Father of Child Care* (Bristol: John Wright and Sons, 1966).

32. Cadogan 1748, 66.

33. Cadogan 1748, 4.

34. Cadogan 1748, 13.

35. Cadogan 1748, 3.

36. Cadogan 1748, 24.

37. See Sussman 1982.

38. See especially his rather self-indulgent ruminations in his *Reveries of a Solitary Walker,* trans. P. France (London: Penguin, 1979), and *Rousseau, Juge de Jean-Jacques* (in

Oeuvres Completes de Jean-Jacques Rousseau, ed. B. Gagnebin and M. Raymond, Paris: Gallimard, Biblotèque de Pléiade, 1959).

39. Quoted in Landes 2001, 98.

40. Quoted in Landes 2001, 98–99.

41. Ivinski et al. 1998, 26.

42. This theme is familiar enough that I have not included a representative image here. For many of them, see especially Landes 2001; Ivinski et al. 1998; and Carol Blum, *Rousseau and the Republic of Virtue* (Ithaca: Cornell University Press, 1986).

43. See Ivinski et al. 1998.

44. Sussman 1982, 110.

45. Yalom 1997, 117.

46. Ivinski et al. 1998, 27.

47. Ivinski et al. 1998, 14.

48. A move that the United States has yet to take!

49. Ivinski et al. 1998, 31.

50. Ivinski et al. 1998, 115.

51. Sussman 1982, 116. Late-eighteenth-century manuals such as P. H. Chavasse, *The Physical Training of Children* (Philadelphia: New World Publishing, 1872) still take it for granted that wet-nursing is one of the major options for infant feeding, although it is usually portrayed as less common than either maternal breastfeeding or feeding with "artificial" infant foods.

52. Kristeva, *Stabat Mater*, trans. A. Goldhammer, in *The Female Body in Western Culture: Contemporary Perspectives*, ed. S. Suleiman (Cambridge, MA: Harvard University Press, 1986), 99–118.

53. Landes 2001, 105.

54. One often-reproduced image of a bare-breasted woman from 1792, by Alexandre Clement after Louis-Simon Boizot, is entitled "La France Republicaine: Ouverant son Sein a tous les Francais," or "Republican France: Opening Her Breast to All the French." See reproductions in both Landes 2001 and Blum 1986.

55. *Emile*, 45.

56. *Emile*, 48.

57. Rousseau, *Confessions*, trans. J. M. Cohen (London: Penguin, 1953), 300–1.

3

Splitting the Maternal Body

In 1809, William Buchan, an English physician who sought to apply Rousseauian principles within the domain of medicine, wrote:

> The more I reflect on the situation of a mother, the more I am struck with the extent of her powers, and the inestimable value of her services. In the language of love, women are called angels; but this is a weak and silly compliment; they approach nearer to our ideas of the Deity: they not only create, but sustain their creation, and hold its future destiny in their hands: every man is what his mother has made him, and to her he must be indebted for the greatest blessing in life, a healthy and a vigorous constitution. . . . But [at the same time] no subsequent endeavors can remedy or correct the evils occasioned by a mother's negligence; and the skill of the physician is exerted in vain to mend what she, through ignorance or inattention, may have unfortunately marred.[1]

Buchan explicitly replaces God with mothers as the producers and designers of human nature. Like God, a mother is capable (with proper discipline) not only of protecting her offspring from unnatural deformity but also of *perfecting* their natures; unlike God, she equally threatens to mar their natures irrevocably, through lapses in her diligence and maternal virtue.

By the early nineteenth century, several of Rousseau's key ideas had been taken up by the French, British, and American medical communities and translated into medical principles. These included the inseparability of physical and moral education and the responsibility of mothers' bodies for building or destroying a well-ordered body politic. What was at stake, in maternal practice, was not just the health of private individuals but also the destiny of the state.[2] Expressing a

65

common early-nineteenth-century refrain, John Abbott wrote, "Mothers have as powerful an influence over the welfare of future generations, as all other causes combined."[3] In the wake of Rousseau, as Michelle Walker puts it, "the mother acts as both guarantor *and* disruptor of man's sociability,"[4] her body promising order, virtue, and unity and equally threatening deformity, depravity, and division. Properly wielded, the maternal body can restore social harmony and stability and inculcate virtue, salving the wounds of a fractured body politic that has fallen away from 'nature.' The improper mother, who fails to breastfeed her child or to discipline her body and her passions, threatens the very constitution of this body politic. Even as the French Revolution used maternal bodies and breasts as symbols of the nurturing and free Republic, it also employed images of female grotesques—ugly and monstrous women with ugly and 'used' breasts—to "materialize the perceived threat of corrupt and disorderly women to the reformed political order."[5] More generally, "women's unlicensed sexuality and untempered enthusiasms were thought to imperil state and civil order."[6] As such, mothers' bodies are appropriate objects of not only medical but also moral and political concern. In an 1816 medical journal, French physician M. F. Billout wrote:

> At all stages of her life, the woman surely inspires the liveliest interest: but does she not present a yet more touching spectacle when, carrying in her breast the promise born of a sacred love, she assures an heir to her family, a citizen of the country! Such a life circumstance merits more attention—*not only the attention of the physician but also that of the politician and the philosopher!*[7]

We saw that in the seventeenth and early eighteenth centuries, mothers' bodies and homes were considered private spaces—inappropriate targets for the gaze of the state or the physician. In the wake of Rousseau, we will see that this reverses quite dramatically. Beginning in the late eighteenth century, mothers' bodies become peculiarly *public* in several senses. Their insides, formerly tucked away behind modesty and ignorance, become objects of rigorous scientific surveillance and attention. Their mundane practices, formerly a matter of private domestic business that the state had little inclination to either aid or regulate, now become a matter of great social import, performed for the public benefit and open to public scrutiny. Accordingly, maternal bodies will now find themselves inserted into the public institutional spaces of professional obstetrics, public benefits programs, anatomy textbooks, family law, and medical education. In a quite concrete sense, the inside of the maternal body will itself be *displaced* into public space through these insertions; Barbara Duden writes of the post-

Revolutionary female body, "Science discovers and professionals control and mediate her womb as a public space. Her flesh becomes the fo-
rum whose proceedings are of immediate interest to the state and society."[8] Along with enormous advances in obstetrical and pediatric
medicine and domestic 'hygiene,' this era would see the first central-
ized systems of financial aid to families and of public health management, as well as sweeping reforms in the organization of foundling
homes and maternity hospitals.

In this chapter, I will be arguing that this insertion and transformation of the maternal body into public space actually splits this body
in two. As it is taken up in imagination and practice in post-
Revolutionary Europe and North America, the maternal body will
now divide into an *unruly*, capricious, improperly and porously
bounded body, easily corrupted and driven by cravings and passions,
and a *fetishized*, well-ordered 'natural' body enjoying perfect unity and
reciprocity with its child. The unruly body needs to be heavily monitored, policed, and regulated in order to keep it from deforming its offspring, while the fetishized body naturally gives birth to virtue, harmony, health, and sociability and needs to be protected from alien
interventions in order to preserve its purity and unity.

ROUSSEAU'S HYSTERICAL DIAGNOSIS

Hysteria was originally the displacement, or the 'wandering,' of the
womb. Through the force of the wayward womb, the reproductive female body supposedly became an incoherent, disorderly space divided
against itself: limbs, eyes, thoughts, and passions no longer work in
concert with one another, but only as capricious fragments.[9] By analogy, a hysterical body politic is also one that is incoherent and divided
against itself, stranded without a general will that can govern all its
parts, in virtue of the improper order and placement of wombs. Hysterical maternal bodies, then, can produce hysterical body politics, according to the post-Rousseauian imagination. At the same time, the
mother who perfects human second nature by keeping her body well-
ordered according to the principles of first nature can heal and prevent
such hysterical social fractures and strengthen and unify the *patrie*.
Medically, hysteria was associated, in the late eighteenth and nineteenth centuries, with women's 'unnatural' cosmopolitan practices:
staying up late, attending the theater, taking up a profession. The traditional cure for hysteria was heterosexual intercourse, marriage, and
childbirth. In normalizing the female reproductive body and regulating
its narrative path, the womb would also purportedly cease its unruly

wanderings and return to its proper place. In turn, normalized maternal bodies were the cure for social hysteria.

Rousseau's own portrayals of the corrupt and fractured body politic regularly trades on images of an incoherent entity whose pieces are fit together inappropriately and artificially, as opposed to forming a seamless, unified whole. The risk of a poor early education, he claims, is that we will be "divided against ourselves,"[10] and "mankind cannot be made by halves."[11] In an "unnatural" society, "swept along in *contrary routes* by nature and by men, forced to *divide ourselves* between these different impulses, we follow a *composite impulse* which leads us to neither one goal nor another. Thus *in conflict and floating* during the whole course of our lives, we end it without having been able to put ourselves *in harmony* with ourselves."[12] *Emile* opens with this principle: "Everything is good as it leaves the hands of the Author of things; everything degenerates in the hands of man. He forces *one soil to nourish the products of another*, one tree to bear the fruit of another. . . . He disfigures everything; he loves deformity, monstrosity."[13] This type of hysterical incoherence, wherein the body (be it individual or politic) becomes a dislocated pastiche of poorly seamed parts, can be taken as the paradigm of the monstrous.[14] Such monstrosity, according to Rousseau, is always a human product, born of our failure to adhere to the unifying principles of first nature

Through this association of *mismatched* sources of nourishment and bearing fruit with deformity, degeneration, and monstrosity, Rousseau lays the ground for figuring wet-nursing, or displaced mothering, as the emblem of this corruption and the nursing of one's own children as its medicine. We will heal hysteria by 'returning' to a state where everything is in its proper, 'natural' place, and the well-ordered bond of maternal milk is the primary medium of this return. "The first education is the most important, and this first education belongs incontestably to women; if the Author of nature had wanted it to belong to men, he would have given them milk with which to nurse children."[15] Only in the wake of Rousseau's dream of the social whole as a natural unity produced and figured by a maternal body could hysteria—division and incoherence caused by a displaced and unruly womb—become such an appropriate imaginative diagnosis of social ills.

Yet at the same time, we will see that the displacement and transformation of the womb into public space became a crucial dimension of the technique for curing these social ills, and hence we can say that hysteria became, in a sense, a prescribed cure for itself. In 1791, Jeremy Bentham published the blueprints for his "Panopticon"—a perfectly transparent and policeable space, designed specifically to house the production of well-ordered and well-harmonized citizen bodies. This genderless, publicly accessible space would make a spectacle out of the formation of human nature, and, Bentham thought, morals would thereby be automatically reformed—indeed, human society would be completely remade *"all by a simple idea in architecture."*[16] Through a spatial transformation, the process of forming human nature could be displaced and publicized, and thereby well-ordered. Bentham in effect proposes a design for a new kind of *reproductive space*: one that will be external and spectacular rather than hidden, ruled by careful engineering principles rather than by a capricious appetitive logic. Throughout this chapter and the next, we will see the Benthamite imagination applied to the maternal body itself.

MONITORING AND MAPPING MATERNAL SPACE

By the nineteenth century, most (though not all) physicians had strictly speaking abandoned the theory of the maternal imagination. However, while rejecting the semiotic character of maternal influences, they retained and even intensified the picture of the maternal body as volatile, permeable, impressionable, and riddled by heightened sensitivities and passions, and of fetal and infant bodies as immediately impacted by the maternal fray. Although the medical establishment would bicker for centuries over whether maternal 'cravings' and 'longings' were to be indulged or denied, there was universal agreement that these irrational drives to ingest were a signal feature of the pregnant body, whose management greatly impacted fetal outcome. But in the post-Rousseauian era, the newfound civic responsibilities of the maternal body turned her permeability, volatility, and immediate impact upon her child into a matter that was inseparably both medical and political. Dr. Fowler writes,

> EVERY CONCEIVABLE state of the maternity affects the embryo. . . . Every pulsation of health in you, will throb through their young veins. Every pang of grief you feel, will leave its painful scar on the forming disk of their souls. Every flash of sweet and pleasurable emotion you experience, will sweeten and beautify, not their conduct merely, but stamp the original impress of amiableness and goodness upon their inmost souls. Every intellectual effort you put forth, will it not render them more thoughtful by nature, the more fond of study, the more clear-headed, contemplative, intelligent and talented? And every exercise of anger, every feeling of temper, every item of crossness and fretfulness in you, at this period, will it not brand this hating and hateful spirit into their inmost souls, to haunt them as long as they exist, here or hereafter? . . . Here, O ye mothers of our race!

> Learn the mighty import of those eventful relations you are compelled to fulfill.[17]

In this passage, maternal passions are still directly transferred onto the bodies of infants, as in earlier centuries, although now the transference is not one of semantic or representational content but of character and capacity—and indeed, it appears that pretty much any maternal state or activity at all can have such direct influence, making the entire maternal body and all its activities into fair game for concern and discipline. Furthermore, a mother's success at controlling her behavior and boundaries has 'import' for the 'race' as a whole and not just for the particular child she bears.

Remember that in the seventeenth century, 'natural' form was a stable benchmark, and a mother's job was to prevent *deforming* her offspring. This meant that as long as a mother protected her fetus or child from deformation, her body had performed its function. But Rousseau, as we saw, upped the bar, introducing a vision of nature as indefinitely improvable. This meant that mothers were capable of not only protecting but also *enhancing* the natures of their offspring. The Rousseauian idea that mothers could positively contribute to fetal development became *medically* viable during the eighteenth century, as new clinical access to and understanding of the insides of the reproductive body disclosed a fetus whose form changed radically during the course of pregnancy, in contrast to the fetus of the seventeenth century representations who began as a fully formed homunculus.

Post-Revolutionary mothers thus came to shoulder a social responsibility for the proper management of their thoughts and motions that in essence had no upper limit. Fowler continues,

> The American and European revolutions are no trifles. Republicanism [will] . . . completely renovate and regenerate society, purging it of all existing evils, political, civil and religious, and prepare our race of a great advance—for a mighty ascent towards heaven. And what we now want is, A CORRESPONDINGLY HIGHER ORDER OF HUMAN BEINGS, TO ENTER UPON THIS PROSPECTIVE GLORY. AND YOU MUST PRODUCE THEM. Oh, what children you could bear, if you knew just how to carry them![18]

Likewise, physician P. H. Chavasse—who, like Buchan and many others, was explicit about his Rousseauian commitments—emphasizes that mothers have not only a negative responsibility to protect their infants but also a positive potential to form great natures; he emphasizes their power to do this during pregnancy and even more through the quality of their milk and through their 'physical training' of infants and young children.[19] Meanwhile, Mrs. C. A. Hopkinson inverts the history of the theory of the maternal imagination, emphasizing the power of mothers' imaginations to improve rather than to deform their offspring: "The ancient Spartan culture, as is well-known, was to hang the rooms of those who were likely to become mothers with pictures of beautiful young men. They believed in the effect of the imagination on the constitution of the child."[20] Notice that while Fowler and Chavasse extend the influence of maternal passions up through childhood, Hopkinson suggests extending it back prior to conception. The need for control over the easily influenced maternal body has thus expanded, by now, to include the whole span of time from preconception through early motherhood and across every dimension of bodily and mental comportment.

Given the heightened civic stake in the comportment of maternal bodies, on the one hand, and their intensified capacity to harm *or* improve, on the other, it is no surprise that these bodies became the object of much more concentrated medical scrutiny and management during the Republican era. Barbara Duden documents how "a good deal of medical writing after 1770 focuses primarily on the discovery, description, and administration of the inner female space from which the 'body politic' had to emerge."[21] In 1788, Wilhelm Ploucquet initiated the technique of palpation, thereby monitoring fetal movements and growth by touching the pregnant woman's belly, breaking longstanding taboos.[22] Ideally, Ploucquet fantasizes, "public baths . . . should be made obligatory" for women of childbearing age so that their pregnancies could be reliably detected.[23] Before the late eighteenth century, the direct examination of the maternal body had been deemed indecent, but from the Revolutionary era onward, the medical penetration and publicization of this maternal body followed a steady march—usually, it should be noted, to the clear medical benefit of women and infants, who had routinely died during childbirth in earlier eras.

One manifestation of this placement of mothers' bodies under the medical eye was the new idea, which did not solidify until near the end of the nineteenth century, that the entire process of pregnancy, childbirth, and child rearing ought to be *monitored* by a physician, even when there was no indication of a special medical problem. We saw that the physician authors of seventeenth-century obstetrical texts designed their works to empower mothers to understand their own bodies and manage their own care. Whereas before the Revolution, physicians were called into the reproductive process only during a medical crisis, in the century after the Revolution it slowly became the mother's *duty* to be overseen by and to obey the prescriptions of a (male) medical professional with a trained eye.[24] Detecting the signs of pregnancy itself became a scientific process that *responsible* would-be mothers must abdicate to a professional. Mrs. Hopkinson advises expectant mothers, "Place yourself at once under the care of your physician. He knows symptoms that you do not. . . . There are various other signs and symptoms of pregnancy, which will not be described, for the reason that it requires an educated physician to detect them and to decide as to their value."[25] Physician oversight—as distinct from physician intervention—gradually became a part of responsible child rearing as well, as 'home remedies' began to get a bad name and texts repeatedly railed against the damage done by nurses and mothers who administered medicines without a physician's supervision and approval. The place of the physician's eye had thus fundamentally transformed since the seventeenth century: the medical gaze went from a daring and dubiously entitled gesture of patient empowerment to a confident expert tribunal of medical assessment. Likewise, the duty of maternal bodily self-governance had also transformed into one that integrally included accountability to medical authority.

The new medical and civic investment in opening up and monitoring maternal space was grounded not solely in the changed moral and political status of mothers' bodies but also in developments within the broader institutions of science and medicine. Foucault points out that "modern medicine has fixed its own date of birth as being in the last years of the eighteenth century," and he famously argues that these years were home to a major overhaul in the epistemological structure of medical practice, as well as in the social and institutional status and organization of the medical profession.[26] On the one hand, it was then that medicine became systematically institutionalized as a profession in a way that put it into close communication and reciprocity with government and state institutions, through public benefits programs, the development of medical jurisprudence,[27] and government oversight of hospitals and medical schools, among other mechanisms. This new professional placement situated medicine as a practice in the service of the *public* good, and not just the good of individual patients, thus "linking medicine with the destinies of states."[28] In turn, Foucault argues, during this era it became the business of medical authorities to regulate civic and domestic life rather than just cure disease—"to punctuate work with festivals, to exalt calm emotions, to watch over what was read in books and seen in theaters, to see that marriages were made not of self-interest or because of a passing infatuation but were based only on the lasting condition of happiness, namely their benefit to the state."[29] Thus "medicine becomes a task for the nation."[30] In other words, professional medicine becomes a bidirectional bridge between the state of individual bodies and the moral and political state of the nation, rather than a private, Hippocratic relationship between a physician and an individual patient.

During these same few decades, Foucault argues, medical examination shifted its focus from the signs and symptoms appearing on the surface of the body to opening and penetrating its inner recesses. The clinic, as an arena in which medical perception could be systematically focused upon individual bodies, became a regulated space with systematic epistemic standards, and touching and dissecting (as opposed to merely observing at the bedside) became the privileged epistemic methods of clinical medicine. In 1801, the celebrated physician and anatomist Marie F. X. Bichat wrote,

> For twenty years, from morning to night, you have taken notes at patients' bedsides on affections of the heart, the lungs, and the gastric viscera, and all is confusion for you in the symptoms which, refusing to yield up their meaning, offer you a succession of incoherent phenomena. Open up a few corpses: you will dissipate at once the darkness that observation alone could not dissipate.[31]

These movements in medicine were by no means restricted to the subspecialties of obstetrics and pediatrics, but they certainly bore a mutually reinforcing relationship to new ideas about the powers and proper treatment of the maternal body. In combination, all these shifts found expression in a systematic deprivatization of the maternal body, both in terms of its suitability as an object to be touched, opened, and penetrated by the scientific gaze and as a subject of social scrutiny and institutional management.

"THE TRUTH WAS THEREBY WELL AUTHENTICATED"

In chapter 1, we saw that prior to the second half of the eighteenth century, medical representations of fetuses and the insides of uteruses were scarce, and those that existed were highly schematic, abstracting the uterus away from the rest of the pregnant body and representing the fetus with the proportions of a grown child. These representational conventions changed dramatically in the second half of the eighteenth century. The break with tradition began with William Smellie, who was arguably the father of modern obstetrics. Smellie's greatest advances were in the use of forceps and other delivery instruments and in the delivery of breech births. His 1754 textbook, *A Theory and Practice of Midwifery*, revolutionized the field and remained the professional standard for decades. Smellie published an accompanying set

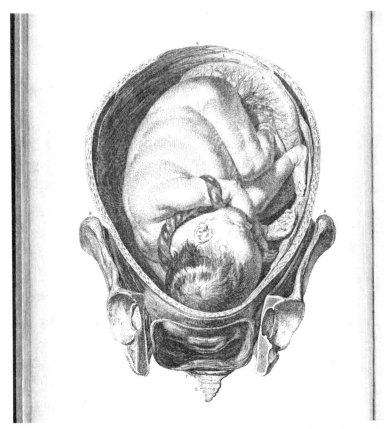

Figure 3.1. William Smellie, *A Set of Anatomical Tables*, Plate IX, 1754, courtesy of the National Library of Medicine.

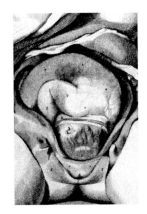

Figure 3.2. Folkert Snip, *Obstetric Observations, and Illustration of a Pregnant Womb*, Plate III, 1767, owned by the Australian and New Zealand College of Obstetricians and Gynecologists, Frank Forster Library, reprinted courtesy of Blackwell Publishing Co.

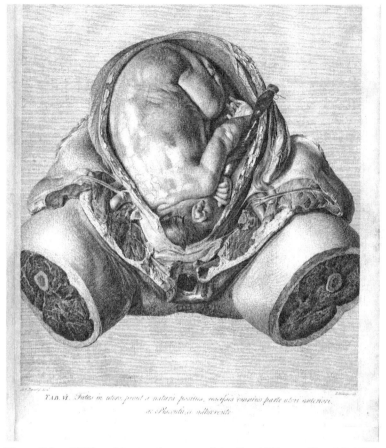

TAB. vi. *Fœtus in utero prout a natura positus, resectis omnino parte uteri anteriori, ac Placenta adhærente*

Figure 3.3.   William Hunter, *Anatomy of the Gravid Uterus*, Plate VI, 1774, courtesy of the National Library of Medicine.

of anatomical plates in tandem with his textbook, and these plates look completely different from any of their predecessors. The plates clearly support and are born out of the new, postprudish, prying medical eye, with its concern for public visibility and objective accuracy. They represent fetuses with careful realism and attention to anatomical and proportional precision. Smellie clearly takes the accurate documentation and display of the normal contents of the womb to be a crucial component of medical teaching and research (see figure 3.1).

However, it was one of Smellie's students, William Hunter, whose anatomical drawings of the pregnant uterus became the new representational standard. In 1774, Hunter published his *Anatomy of the Human Gravid Uterus*—a glorious set of plates displaying an unprecedented fidelity to detail. Hunter hired an artist to document his dissections of deceased women at various stages of pregnancy. He dissected the women layer by layer, documenting each stage, so that the plates move successively inward from just under the surface of the skin, through the uterine wall, through the amniotic sac, to the fetus itself. Smellie was concerned to represent the exact proportions of his subjects, but he was willing to leave out details in order to heighten the illustrative clarity of his drawings. Hunter, on the other hand, considered *any* dropped detail a betrayal of his subject, and consequently his drawings display an excruciating level of mimetic realism. His commitment to perfect naturalistic representation of his subjects was so great that he insisted that the drawings be exactly life-sized so that not even their dimensions would be distorted by the representational process. The plates are almost overwhelming to witness in the original, and their enormity certainly contributes to their sublime character.

Hunter's plates depart from Smellie's in another important way as well. Despite his concern with naturalism, Smellie continued the convention of abstracting the uterus away from the body of the pregnant woman in which it was housed; his uteruses are crisply bounded spaces suspended against a white background. In 1767, in between the publication of Smellie's plates and Hunter's, the Dutch obstetrician Folkert Snip placed the uterus back into the female body (see figure 3.2). Snip's drawings do not have the detail of Hunter's, but by offering naturalistic representations of the entire dissected female torso (with the "private parts" delicately covered with a sheet), they make explicit the new medical access to the inside of women's bodies—access that is still visually elided in Smellie's plates. However Hunter, unlike any of his predecessors, not only visually acknowledged his access to women's bodies but also applied his high standards of detailed mimetic representation to the entirety of the body he dissected. Far from modestly protecting maternal bodies from the public eye, Hunter represents every fleshy contour of the bodies that he has literally butchered for the occasion. The cut torso of his pregnant subject is represented as ragged and bloody around the edges where its limbs have been sawed off. Its skin and vagina, mutilated for the purposes of maximal visual access, are displayed in all their wounded specificity. His maternal bodies are just flesh. He willfully excises any trace of embarrassment or shame that might interrupt his images, remaining true to his goal of representing the uterus and its contents completely and accurately, in their proper bodily and scientific context (see figure 3.3). In the same year that Hunter published his plates, Jacques Fabien Gautier d'Agoty also planted the naturalistically represented fetus back into the fleshy female body. His drawings could never be accused of mimetic realism, given that his female subjects have transparent ab-domens, no skin, and are not only very much alive but quite calm in the face of their predicament. Yet d'Agoty forces our shameless ac-knowledgment of the agent in whom gestation occurs by having his pregnant subject look us directly in the eye while she publicly displays her insides (see cover illustration).

William Hunter—who also conducted a series of experiments de-signed to scientifically debunk the theory of the maternal imagina-tion[32]—was quite conscious of his status as an epistemic and not just a technical pioneer. Proper opportunities for dissecting pregnant women were few and far between, he notes in his preface. But luckily for him, "A young woman died suddenly, when very near the end of pregnancy. The body was prepared before any sensible putrefaction had begun. The season of the year was favourable for dissection, the in-jection of the blood vessels proved very successful; a very able painter, in this way, was found. Every part was examined *in the most public manner, and the truth was thereby well-authenticated.*" Hence, he continues, he has succeeded in producing an image that "represents what was actually seen, it carries the *mark of truth*, and becomes al-most as infallible as the object itself."[33] This explicit commitment to complete fidelity to the object as a regulative ideal, and to *publicity* as a crucial element of scientific authority and verification, is new to ob-stetrics. Hunter's understanding of the authentication of truth is actu-ally quite complex—he is exceptionally willing to intervene upon the body for the purposes of opening it up and displaying its insides, but interestingly, he does not count this intervention as a distortion or a transformation of that body. His caption to figure 3.3 reads in part, "Every part is represented just as it was found; not so much as one joint of a finger having been moved to shew any part more distinctly, or to give a more picturesque effect."[34] Thus the *opening* of the body does not count, for him, as an alteration of that body but rather as a tool for the proper unmediated observation of it—the normally closed skin of the female body is now what distorts proper vision.

This new visual publicity of the pregnant body arose alongside two new genres of texts about pregnancy and early motherhood, both sharply distinguished from the reasonably unified corpus of early mod-ern texts I examined in chapter 1. Both of these new genres gave ex-pression to the changing scientific and social place of mothers' bodies.

On the one hand, there emerged a corpus of obstetrical textbooks, spearheaded by Smellie's *Treatise on Midwifery*. Smellie's textbook manifested a radical break from the works I examined in chapter 1, not only in content but also in style and voice. The text is addressed to fel-low (male) obstetrical students and practitioners, rather than to female patients, and it presumes the presence of a male physician during labor. Accordingly, these patients show up in the text as objects of medical study and management, rather than as an audience for the book in a dialogical relationship with its author. The text matter-of-factly divides the female body into parts for independent examination, and it includes detailed sections on the proper techniques for touching and penetrating female patients with fingers and instruments, during internal exams and during labor. A large set of books over the next century followed closely in Smellie's footsteps, mimicking the structure and voice of his work. These works adopted a carefully dispassionate, scientific, and at least apparently value-free language and used it to dissect and describe the female reproductive body, along with the most current techniques for its medical management.[35] The intimate and daring tone of the seventeenth-century texts is noticeably absent in these works; the second-person voice has been replaced by passive constructions, wherein states of the reproductive body "are observed."

Even a cursory look at these texts makes it clear that, in the interim since Mauriceau, Sadler, Culpeper, and their peers were writing, an entire institution of professional and academic medical obstetrics has been established. These new works are—proudly—not private handbooks for women but rather professional *tools*. Smellie is particularly vitriolic, in his preface, toward Culpeper, whose bawdy and personal style Smellie finds offensively unprofessional, suited only to the "lower sort" with "weak heads."[36] Several of these modern obstetricians comment upon the morbidity and mortality that has been caused by ignorant, prudish resistance to the medically trained (male) surveillance of pregnancy and birth. All of these writers treat internal exams and regular attendance at birth by male physicians as a given, routine dimension of obstetrical care (although in fact this was not nearly as routine at the time as they make it sound in their texts). They also all discuss the indications and techniques for using instruments to artificially intervene in labor. They go out of their way not to speak prudishly or euphemistically about the female body, and the texts are often graphically illustrated. The chapters on monstrous and false births, ubiquitous in earlier centuries, are completely absent now, and in their place are standardized sections on the routine diseases and discomforts of normal pregnancy (heartburn, morning sickness, and the like). Written for physicians and from a physician's point of view, these works devote little or no time to the regulation of maternal lifestyle, sticking instead to anatomical and clinical details.

Coincident with this birth of the modern professional obstetrical textbook, there emerged a distinct set of works written as advice books for mothers. Also written by physicians, these were the precursors to *Dr. Spock's Baby and Child Care* and *What to Expect When You're Expecting*, as opposed to *Williams Obstetrics*.[37] These books advised women on how to conduct themselves and care for their bodies during pregnancy, childbirth, and early motherhood. Whereas the professional texts break the maternal body into layers and sections, these texts address themselves to the lifestyle and narrative of the maternal body as a whole. They are generally written in the second rather than the third person, resuming the intimate address of the seventeenth-century texts, although with none of the earlier tones of privacy or political daring. The guides are as suffused with normative language as the medical textbooks are excised of it. Self-consciously weaving together moral and medical advice into a tight unity, they portray the care of mothers' and infants' bodies as a project that is at every turn governed by principles of duty, virtue, and religious and social obligation.

Maternal duties, in these guidebooks, are sacred duties laid down by God, nature, and nation, and the proper regulation and governance of the body is the primary terrain of these duties. They each contain a multitude of mundane recommendations for this regulation and governance, with elaborate routines for feeding, dressing, sleeping, exercising, and otherwise managing both mothers' and infants' bodies. While they diverge in the details, their general messages are shared. These are: (1) Pregnant women and new mothers must "subdue every passion,"[38] for passions are communicated directly to the child and will corrupt its character. Mothers must be unendingly vigilant in their self-control, policing their passions and boundaries, because (these books agree) the pre- and postnatal body is especially volatile and susceptible to nervous and imaginative excesses and imbalances. (2) Mothers are not only *capable* of deforming their children but also *morally responsible* for doing so through insufficient discipline over their own bodies. Fowler, who, interestingly, was one of the most prominent promoters of phrenology, writes, "If our women would follow the advice given in the preceding sections, . . . they would seldom mark their children, because they themselves would seldom be impressed with these foreign influences, but would generally resist them."[39] And of the bad-tempered, problematic child, he comments, "He is but the passive agent. Suppose you punish the REAL cause—YOUR OWN SELF."[40] (3) In regulating her body, the expectant or new mother ought to be governed by the laws of 'nature,' where natural laws are inherently normative and prescriptive rather than mechanistic and descriptive. Like Cadogan and Rousseau, the authors of these guides take first nature as providing principles that properly govern the formation of second natures. Nature is the guide to proper maternal practice, and "Nature's laws cannot be broken without impunity."[41]

Following Rousseau, these works regularly cite the use of 'artificial' medicines, fashionable clothing, urban as opposed to 'peasant' or 'savage' lifestyles, and especially mothers' failure to breastfeed their own children as examples of practices that betray the maternal laws of nature. The *proximity* of the child to the mother's breast is often elevated into an incarnation of the tight natural unity and order that was supposed to govern the relationship between mother and infant. In the name of following nature, there was a movement among early-nineteenth-century physicians to divert funding away from foundling hospitals toward direct aid for low-income families so as to promote mother-infant proximity and maternal breastfeeding.[42] Walter Coles writes that the maternal "breast is *nature's medicine*" and warns that interrupting this physical bond between mother and child with artificial medicines and foods or other interventions will corrupt them both: "A sensible, well-informed nurse will readily appreciate the importance of leaving the baby to nature, and of compelling it to swallow nothing but what it obtains in the natural way from its mother."[43] In an explicitly Rousseauian voice, Dr. Buchan claims that while European mothers are deforming their children through their use of artificial medicines, foods, and instruments, North American "savages" have no deformed children at all because "they never thwart the purposes of nature, or disobey her dictates, in the treatment of their infant progeny."[44]

That there should be these two kinds of texts—dry professional medical textbooks that aspire to be 'value-free' and objective, on the one hand, and chatty guidebooks for mothers driven by normative visions of proper maternality, on the other—is not surprising, as both genres are alive and well. Indeed, if anything is remarkable about these 200-year-old texts, it is how similar they are from their contemporary complements, in tone, style, and even broad-strokes content—as we will see more clearly when we turn to these contemporary works in subsequent chapters. But it is important to see how this textual division of labor is a historical product. The pre-Revolutionary works on pregnancy combined the functions of both genres, covering both the clinical and the dietetic dimensions of reproduction, and were distinct from either of them in both voice and content. The decoupling of these two genres was a late-eighteenth-century event that had among its preconditions substantial shifts in the politics of maternal bodies; the institution of the welfare state; changes in our conceptions of nature, personhood, and virtue; and major scientific and professional advancements in medicine.

THE FETISH MOTHER AND THE UNRULY MOTHER

Over the course of this book so far, I have pointed out ways in which our picture of the maternal body and its powers and responsibilities is double-edged; this picture elicits anxieties over its power to deform, as well as romantic admiration for its power to restore, perfect, and harmonize nature. Dr. Buchan writes, "everything is perfect, says Rousseau, as it comes out of the hands of God; but everything degenerates in the hands of man. This is particularly true of the human species. . . . What a train of ills seems to await the precious charge, the moment it is taken out of the hands of nature! But as the most of these calamities are the consequences of [mothers'] mismanagement or neglect, I shall endeavor to show how they may be prevented by tended and rational attention."[45] Maternal practice is responsible for the corruption of nature and order, and equally the hope of their restoration. Now I want to argue that beginning in the late eighteenth century, these two sides of our imaginative grasp of maternal bodies led to the birth of two distinct imaginary mother figures, and that these two figures shaped the modern care, practices, and understanding of actual mothers' bodies in Europe and North America. In part II of this book, I will argue that these two maternal figures continue to exert a powerful and formative influence over the institutions surrounding motherhood and the practices and care of individual women.

These two maternal bodies or figures are not, of course, literal bodies, but neither are they mere symbols or archetypes or myths. Rather, they are idealized, imaginary bodies through which we read, interpret, negotiate, and judge mothers' actual bodies (whether these are our own bodies or not). Our care and treatment of maternal (and fetal and infant) bodies is *animated* by these two maternal figures; this applies both to the concrete care of these bodies as medical patients and as citizens within a social system, and to the representation of these bodies as cultural symbols and subjects. Crucially, the *interaction* between these two figurative bodies—the ways in which they complement, constitute, and contradict one another—is itself a major animator of the concrete narratives of real, particular maternal bodies. Though the two bodies appear in various ways to be contraries, I will argue that they are necessary complements or even supplements of one another, born out of the same set of late Enlightenment ideas, practices, and concerns that we have already been examining in detail. Out of the post-Rousseauian reconstitution of maternality and its relationships to medicine and to the state emerged what I will name the "Fetish Mother" and the "Unruly Mother."

A *fetish* is an object perceived as having inherent normative value and power, where this normative status (apparently) attaches to the object as an atomic, independent whole rather than as a product of its context or its internal compositional structure. A fetishized commodity, for instance, is one whose desirability and value appear intrinsic to the object itself, independent of the vectors of supply and demand, production, marketing, or need.[46] Fetishes are ahistorical; they present themselves to us as primary *sources* of value and desire rather than as historically generated products of them. The internal workings and the history of a fetish are never an explicit part of the ideology that supports it; this ideology will appeal to the fetish to explain value, rather than the other way around.[47] In general, fetishes appear to bridge the problematic gap between 'is' and 'ought'—they are objects that are experienced as having value built into their very essence. Freud extended this basic Marxian account of fetishization to the domains of sexuality and religion: a sexual fetish is an object experienced as immediately and independently erotically desirable, and a religious fetish is taken as inherently divine. A crucial feature of fetishes is that their value and power are not products of the values and powers of their parts. A foot fetishist is not generally seduced by the sum of a disjointed set of toes, nor is a Mercedes fetishist seduced by a Mercedes carburetor, except perhaps insofar as these parts get their meaning through their synecdochal association with the whole, rather than the other way around.

My claim is that the 'natural' maternal body, and especially the body of the nursing mother, can be productively interpreted as functioning as a *social* fetish in post-Revolutionary Western culture—that is, it is experienced as an inherent, atomic source of social (as opposed to economic, sexual, or divine) value and power. Her body is a perfect and uninterrupted whole, which includes the body of her fetus or infant. The Fetish Mother enjoys an uninterrupted 'natural' unity with her child. The *space* of her body includes her infant, which begins inside of her and is then sutured to her naturally through her breast and its milk. The surface of her body is a public spectacle symbolizing the possibility of well-ordered human nature free from hysterical incoherence, artificial hybrids, or deformed monstrosity.

As emblematic of nonhysterical society, the Fetish Mother is figured as seamlessly bonded with her child in a way that makes no room for internal articulation or division. Her body is itself inherently nonhysterical, as she does not allow her child to be displaced from its proper site, and she is not fractured by any artificial interruptions or deformations. The performative power of this image of natural unity without seams was an important corrective to the Rousseauian suspicion that second natures could only be at best contingently harmonized. The proper maternal body is not supposed to return us to first nature, but she is supposed to bestow upon us the seamless unity that first nature supposedly had before it was butchered by society and reassembled into a mismatched, fractured union. It is no accident that the female figure of liberty stood, in the French Republic, specifically for the freedom enabled by an *undivided* society. Indeed, the Fetish Mother is capable of fulfilling what Foucault calls one of the "dreams" of the Revolutionary and post-Revolutionary era, namely that society can be reordered through the proper care of the bodies of its citizens and thereby "restored to its original state of health."[48] This is the work cut out for her body by Rousseau, and it inherently involves this nostalgic turn to first nature as the normative tribunal of second nature.

As long as artificial forces don't interrupt its perfect natural order, this body will produce well-ordered nature. Thus it must be protected from 'unnatural' penetrations and interventions—such as physicians' fingers, artificial medicines, and wet nurses—that can create a schism in the unity of the body, opening the door to disorder and hysteria. In contrast, the wet nurse and the infant she suckles will always be an artificial conglomerate of two naturally separate beings. As such, the wet nurse is a monstrous figure, a deceptive simulacra of the natural, extended maternal body, while the unnatural mother who voluntarily severs her proximity from her infant and sends it out to nurse is the agent of this monstrous separation. Dr. Buchan comments, "If we take a view of all animated nature, it is shocking to find, that woman should be the only monster capable of withholding the nutritive fluid from her young. Such a monster, however, does not exist among savage nations."[49]

Not surprisingly, the Fetish Mother is never successfully incarnated in her pure form; she serves instead as a regulative ideal governing the proper principles of maternal nourishment and care. Joan Landes points out that in contrast to the many portraits of the fathers of the French Revolution that were used as public icons, the nursing and bare-breasted figures used to represent the Republic and its virtues were never modeled after any particular women; Marianne, she reminds us, is only a picture.[50] The Fetish Mother exists as a *guiding image* of appropriate motherhood, which at the same time expresses the purported essence of 'true' maternality.

In contrast, the Unruly Mother is a volatile, fragile, contingent, appetitive being, with little resistance against temptation, craving, and the extremities of passion. She is governed not by orderly principles but by an ad hoc, capricious logic of sentiment and craving. Easily penetrated, she must be carefully regulated, policed, and controlled, for her disorderly nature is always at risk of hysteria,[51] and this hysteria is highly contagious—it will deform her offspring and through them transmit itself to the body politic. Her powers are no less than those of the Fetish Mother, but she cannot be trusted to carry out her enormous social and moral responsibilities without oversight and governance. The spaces of her body and home must be relocated to the public domain and rendered panoptic so as to make them manageable by responsible, more stable social and scientific institutions. Through such public discipline and surveillance, the Unruly Mother will hopefully be prevented from inappropriately ingesting things, leaking things, and unnaturally disordering and separating that which ought to remain harmonized and unified.

Pregnancy "especially exposes [women] to the agency of external and noxious impressions and mental emotions," and pregnant women thus purportedly tend toward being "disordered" and "thrown off their balance."[52] Combined with the unnatural temptations and practices of modern cosmopolitan life, this heightened vulnerability left the womb and home of the modern, post-Revolutionary pregnant woman especially open to deforming corruption. Modern society encouraged and gratified women's appetites and enthusiasms, stirred their passions, and penetrated their already fragile boundaries with poisons. It also further weakened these boundaries, since mothers of a "nervous and delicate constitution . . . who have always been accustomed to having their wishes gratified, and who all their lives have had nothing to think about—but themselves,"[53] were the ones supposedly most prone to unruly cravings and least able to exercise control over them. In Fleetwood Churchill's generally dispassionate medical textbook on the diseases of women, he sharply criticizes his society's encouragement of the "unlimited gratification" of pregnant women's "depraved" appetites, and he lists cases where this gratification purportedly led to the deformity or death of the fetus. Thus, he argues, these women "should not be allowed to indulge in all the capriciousness and wanton absurdities of their appetites."[54]

The excesses of modern life supposedly deformed not only women's mental states but also their literal shapes as well: many works of the era contain elaborate descriptions and drawings of deformed wombs and pelvises blamed on urban clothes and lifestyles.[55] The focus on pelvises and wombs in particular made vivid the idea that women were deforming the *space of reproduction* itself through their hysterical behavior. In a remarkable little late-nineteenth-century volume, Dr. J. C. Petit, M.D., advises the sales-ladies in his employ on how to market his personal invention, the "womb battery," through parlor gatherings that were apparently structured like twentieth-century Tupperware parties. He billed the womb battery as a device that would "fix" the womb and thereby cure all "women's diseases." The device was in fact an electric dildo that "worked" by giving women orgasms—upon application, "she will feel a delicious chill course through her whole being." According to Petit, disorders of the womb were on the rise because the health of the womb was "degenerating" as women became "freer and more accomplished" and "entered various professions." The womb battery, Petit writes, "destroys every germ of disease lurking in the creative receptacle of the female sex. . . . If your body is a physical wreck, your offspring are a curse to themselves and the world and a misnomer to motherhood. . . . With [this device] in her possession she is enabled to control at will, and become a heavenly blessing to herself and family."[56]

Mothers were implored to develop self-control and self-discipline in order to compensate for their vulnerable and poorly bounded bodies. Although their propensity to cravings and disorder were taken as given facts about the nature of their reproductive bodies, these propensities could be controlled with proper dedication. "Can a mother expect to govern her child, when she cannot govern herself? . . . She must learn to control herself; to subdue her own passions," John Abbott entreats.[57] But the control and discipline of maternal bodies was an appropriate responsibility for external authorities as well. Whereas in seventeenth-century texts physicians warned mothers to protect their imaginations from stimulation and to regulate their bodies, by the nineteenth century physicians saw this protection and regulation as part of their professional responsibility—'border control' now fell under the scope of their authority. Churchill writes, "The diet must be carefully regulated; on the one hand *we may allow* a reasonable indulgence to the patient's taste, but on the other, inordinate or capricious fancies must be opposed. . . . All external excitements should be carefully shunned."[58]

The Fetish Mother is a romantic, idealized character, while the Unruly Mother is an object of distrust and disdain. The first needs protection from external interventions, while the latter needs external interventions for proper discipline and management. Both, however, are born of the idea that the maternal body is responsible for the production of human and social nature, properly governed by normative laws of nature, and easily corrupted and interrupted. Both maternal bodies enjoy an exceptionally tight relationship with infant bodies, whether this relationship is one of romantic unity or of the transmittal of disorder. Both bodies are peculiarly public, although in nearly opposite ways: Where the Fetish Mother functions as a public spectacle symbolizing and creating natural order, the Unruly Mother's body needs to be displaced into public space so that it can be prevented from spreading hysteria and unnatural disorder. The half-naked *surface* of the body of the

Fetish Mother proudly adorned public monuments, books, and visual propaganda, serving as a symbol for exalted virtues such as liberty, truth, and equality. At the same time, the *inside* of the Unruly Mother's body was a different kind of public spectacle, carefully displayed in anatomy books and surgical theaters. Meanwhile, both bodies have nontraditional boundaries: The body of the Fetish Mother extends to encompass her infant-citizens, while the body of the Unruly Mother is doubly permeable, open to the disordering influences of passions and poisons and rendered transparent to the regulatory eye of medicine and the state. The Fetish Mother's nontraditional boundaries also find an important precedent in earlier figures of maternality; in its pure form, the Fetish Mother is *immaculate*—sealed off and joined seamlessly with her infant, whose creation and sustenance involve no puncturing of her borders. Such an image of immaculate motherhood obviously predates any Enlightenment picture of mothers as the guarantors of the humanistic, secular body politic. But in the wake of Rousseau, this image comes to stand for the undivided and unruptured social whole whose integrity she is charged with birthing and nourishing. Both sets of nontraditional boundaries are special sites for social anxiety: the boundaries of the Unruly Mother must be regulated and controlled, whereas those of the Fetish Mother must be protected from violation. It is to this latter set of anxieties that I turn in the next section.

DISSECTING MONSTERS

At the same time as medical obstetrics was developing as a professionalized field, in the business of improving maternal and fetal outcomes through the penetration and display of the insides of maternal bodies, a vocal countermovement vigorously opposed these professional developments. A series of texts published from the late eighteenth through the mid-nineteenth century criticized the new involvement of professional male obstetricians in childbirth and labor. It is important to note right off the bat that these critiques were themselves also based in a male medical community—one with rather traditional, conservative ideas about gender roles. Although a small number of women did contribute to the debate, for the most part this was a debate among gentlemen concerning the proper care and handling of maternal bodies.

The critique of the male obstetricians was most visibly articulated by John Blunt, Philip Thicknesse, and Samuel Gregory, in a series of polemics that garnered quite a bit of public attention.[59] In the middle of the eighteenth century, Dr. Smellie had influentially argued not only that male obstetricians had a proper place in the medical management of pregnancy and birth but also, perhaps more significantly, that normal, healthy pregnancies should receive ongoing professional medical oversight. Smellie thought that the prior practice of involving physicians only during medical emergencies, when they would be brought in to treat a patient with whose history and situation they were unfamiliar, was based in ignorance and prudery. Smellie and his followers[60] quickly became the explicit, ad hominem target for the opponents of such modern obstetrical practices.

While the physicians who took up the specialty of managing reproduction usually referred to themselves as "accoucheurs," their critics called them "man-midwives," which is a term that makes no appearance in professional obstetrical textbooks. The term already marks what critics saw as the unnatural, monstrous character of the enterprise. The man-midwife transgressed a natural boundary between the genders, thereby transforming himself into a hybrid being who, like unnatural mothers, would beget monstrosity out of his own monstrosity. We have seen attempts to regulate the body of the Unruly Mother in order to prevent her from creating monstrosity from *within*; the crusade against the man-midwife was born of the symmetrical fear that unnatural and unruly doctors would create monstrosity by penetrating and disordering maternal bodies from the *outside*. Left to follow nature, critics claimed, the maternal body would produce well-ordered offspring, families, and nations. Unnatural doctors supposedly jeopardized the order of all three. Through medical malpractice they assaulted and deformed infant bodies; through assaults on the modesty and decency of mothers they deformed families; through transgressions of natural boundaries between genders and professions they deformed the social order itself.

What most interests me about the critique of man-midwifery is the surprising fact that its primary concern was not, as one might have guessed, the general indecency of men prying into women's private parts. Rather, the critique was very specifically focused, in the first instance, on the greater propensity of male obstetricians (as opposed to midwives) to use *instruments* to *penetrate and pierce* the bodies of pregnant and laboring women. It is the 'cutting' and 'tearing' of the maternal body, and through it the infant body, that resurfaces as the primary source of monstrosity in every text critiquing man-midwives. By using female midwives, John Blunt claims, "husbands may INFALLIBLY prevent the tearing of their wives and the cutting of their children."[61] Man-midwives were perceived as *professional dissectors* of maternal and infant bodies, just as dissection was becoming an acceptable tool of obstetrical knowledge. Critics saw the dissection of live, 'natural' pregnant bodies as an assault that transgressed the proper boundaries of these bodies. Indeed, the indecency of this penetration and piercing across gender lines and its sexual connotations are invariably introduced as both causally and rhetorically derivative upon the more basic problem of the overuse of artificial instruments during labor. Men in the business of penetrating women with instruments would supposedly show less restraint when it came to penetrating their patients with instruments of a fleshier and old-fashioned sort, and women who got used to being so penetrated would be aroused and made more receptive to immoral advances.

None of the polemics claim that it is the gender of the man-midwives *per se* that makes their attendance at births inappropriate. Rather, it is the ethos of professional obstetrics that comes under attack, although this ethos is clearly perceived as deeply gendered, shaped by male professional ambition and a guiding desire to supplant womanly nature with manly science. The artificial cutting and piercing of the maternal body is portrayed, in these texts, as an urge or a *craving* of the man-midwife, a temptation at the level of the body that is eerily akin to the cravings that characterize the pregnant body itself; male obstetricians were warned to take steps to control and police their own irrational temptations, much as were their pregnant patients. Dr. James Blundell, an obstetrician himself and one of the few moderates in this debate, writes coyly, "Some men seem to have a sort of instinctive impulse to put the lever or the forceps into the vagina. Repeatedly I shall state to you, that you are not needlessly to interfere with the natural efforts. It is only, therefore, in those cases where you have every reason to expect difficulty, that you are justified in taking your instruments. Lead yourself not into temptation; if you put your instruments into your pocket, they are very apt to slip out of your pocket and into the uterus."[62]

In the last section, I argued that the Fetish Mother was demarcated by her freedom from artificial interruptions, separations, and penetrations; her sealed boundaries and unity are the purported source of her normative status and power. Even as Europe was learning to penetrate the unruly maternal body in order to protect the reproductive process, then, this development was offset by a countermovement that feared alien violations and penetrations of the fetishized maternal body.

This countermovement can quite precisely be counted as the beginning of the modern 'natural childbirth' movement—a beginning, I stress again, that sprung from a desire to preserve traditional gender roles and maintain the marginalization of women's health care, and a romantic fetishization of pregnancy and birth, all seated in a community of male physicians and conservative social critics (and *not* a community of radical feminist midwives or female patients). We saw that in the seventeenth century, 'natural' births were counted as those in which an undeformed fetus was in the normal, head-down position at the onset of labor. Unnatural births posed a medical challenge, but they were not especially morally significant. During the second half of the eighteenth century, the definition of a 'natural birth' explicitly shifted to one that did not involve the alien interruption of penetration of the laboring body with instruments or other 'artificial' interventions.[63] In the hands of the critics of man-midwifery, 'natural childbirth,' or childbirth that was completed without such alien influence, took on a normative and even a moral valence very similar to what it has now; it came to be read as a preservation of the body of the Fetish Mother and hence a protection of proper maternality and the natural law.

According to critics, 'nature' is almost always sufficient for delivering a baby safely, but male obstetricians interrupt and pervert this natural process as a matter of professional routine. The obstetricians supposedly seek to *displace* nature as the governor of the maternal body. The anti-man-midwifery polemics are each peppered with anecdotes such as the following, designed to demonstrate the negligent, arrogant, and damaging zeal of man-midwives to supplant nature and to violate and penetrate natural maternal bodies with alien instruments:

> The following story is a matter of fact, which happened lately in the West of England. A . . . man-midwife, being sent for in great haste to deliver a woman, did, as soon as he arrived, in order I suppose to show his dexterity, by the means of a Hook, deliver her instantly from her pain, and the child from a life, it could scarcely be said to have enter'd into, and having so done, took his fee and his leave; but before he had got two miles off, he was pursued and overtaken by the Husband, who desired his immediate return, as the pains of his wife were come on again in a more violent manner than every; but before the husband and doctor got back, she was delivered of another child, by the help *only* of that excellent, and never failing female midwife, Goody Nature! This old lady . . . was, about fifty years ago, stifled in France between two feather-beds. . . ; no sooner was the good old lady interred, than . . . male impostors in that fantastical country, endeavored to intrude themselves on the public as her legitimate sons; nay, to be able by their art, and with the help of hooks, crotchets, fillets, forceps, and scissors, to surpass the good old lady.[64]

Male obstetricians were portrayed as sadistically and stubbornly bent on using instruments on their patients, for reasons of professional pride and hubris along with the sexual and violent proclivities inherent to their gender and their vocation: "Surgeons are very improper persons, to attend natural labours, being too familiar with instruments, and insensible to human pain."[65] Smellie himself defensively acknowledges this perception: "A general outcry has been raised against gentlemen of the profession, as if they *delighted* in using instruments and violent methods in the course of their practice."[66]

The frontispiece to Blunt's aptly named *Man-Midwifery Dissected* is frequently reprinted and cited as emblematic of the debate (see figure 3.4). The rich and memorable image shows a hybrid human figure whose right half is a male obstetrician and whose left half is a female midwife. The female side of the picture is drawn in soft, flowing lines that taper off and almost disappear as the picture gets symbolically closer to the laboring woman's body. The midwife is ushering out the child with a gesture; her hand, stretching outward toward her implied patient, suggests service to the maternal body rather than any proprietary stance toward it or invasion of it. The ground is soft and the fire behind her inviting. The space into which her patient will presumably give birth is a vessel for the new extension of the maternal body, and it does not threaten to intrude. In contrast, the male half of the picture is drawn in sharp, bold lines. The male doctor is surrounded by tools and instruments that are literally designed to pierce the maternal body: huge 'boring scissors' with vicious blades, forceps, an enormous hook, a lever, and shelf upon shelf of medications and potions. Clearly the birth he is attending will be heavily mediated by the artificial manipulations of the medical profession, and this doctor has no intention of protecting the sealed boundaries of the maternal body. Even the floor on his side of the picture is a triumph of artifice over nature; clean lines and corners suggest hard planed boards. One shelf of potions is labeled "this shelf for my own use." The label marks the explicit separateness of the male physician from his female patient, as

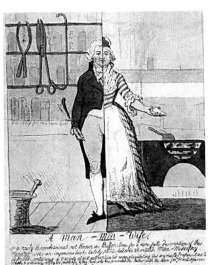

Figure 3.4. Frontispiece, John Blunt, *Man-Midwifery Dissected*, 1993, courtesy of the Countway Medical Library at Harvard University.

well as his membership in a profession that protects the turf of its trade and has special technical 'insiders' knowledge. The male hand points inward, toward the doctor rather than toward the presumed patient. It wields a sharp object ready to be used at a moment's notice. The split structure of the picture as a whole not only contrasts the two kinds of births and birth attendants but also represents the man-midwife himself as a hybrid creature, an unnatural monster hysterically fragmented, born of science and male ambition rather than nature, just as the children he delivers will be.

This vision of a male drive to displace nature and co-opt the maternal body, to create monsters who are cut and sewn into unnatural, hysterical figures rather than natural, unified beings with sealed boundaries, and even the slippage between the fractured monstrosity of the beings *born* of such masculine ambitions and interventions and the fractured monstrosity of the man-midwife himself, are—it need hardly be said—familiar to us. In 1818, in the midst of the obstetrical revolution and its backlash, Mary Shelley published *Frankenstein, or a Modern Prometheus*, a work in which she "endeavored to preserve the truth of the elementary principles of human nature."[67] Surely the novel both captured and formed our shared imagination of birth, nature, and monstrosity to an extent rarely surpassed in human history. Conceived and set in Rousseau's Geneva, and written during Shelley's pregnancy, the novel's protagonist, Victor Frankenstein, is an ambitious young scientist who "conceives" of his monster at the same age as Shelley "conceived" both her child and her novel, namely nineteen. Dr. Frankenstein is both her double and her alter-ego. Like any pregnant woman, he possesses the creative power to generate life and the terrifying power to deform it. But Frankenstein's creation works against and over nature rather than through it. His monster is no part of him; indeed he rejects it and thrusts it into solitude. *Frankenstein* can be read as expressing twin anxieties surrounding the maternal body at the time. The parable as a whole expresses the recurring motifs of the dangers of human generation that thwarts rather than follows nature, that creates pastiches rather than well-ordered wholes, and that separates the body of the child from its creator. At the same time, Victor Frankenstein's specific gender, profession, and ambition turn the story into a narrative critique of the dangers of man-midwifery and the male lust to co-opt birth.[68]

This dream of the masculine temptation to supplant nature as the director and designer of human generation, and the threat of hysterical disorder and monstrous hybridism that are embedded in this dream, have found expression again and again since Rousseau and Shelley crystallized them in our imagination. In 1896, H. G. Wells' Dr. Moreau, a vivisectionist chased out of England for his inappropriate dissections, would try to make humans out of animals, transforming the capricious brute into a "rational creature of my own."[69] But, he discovers, the "beast always creeps back in,"[70] and instead of rationalizing nature he produces untamable hybrid monsters, doomed to be collections of pieces rather than unified wholes. Dr. Frankenstein's secret laboratory and Dr. Moreau's remote island are themselves displaced wombs emblematic of hysteria. In the early twentieth century, we continued to be compelled by and afraid of the same dream, fixated on (what are still mere) fantasies of genetically engineered and enhanced and cloned humans—products of scientific planning rather than uninterrupted natural maternal unfolding, generated in spaces of reproduction displaced from the proper maternal body. Our imaginative fascination with these fantasies and our gut sense that such creatures would be monstrous disruptors of the natural order have largely supplanted any careful critical discourse concerning the public health advantages and disadvantages of pursuing the relevant technology.[71]

BODIES BORDERING ON THE PATHOLOGICAL

Fleetwood Churchill reminds the readers of his treatise on the diseases of pregnancy and childbirth that both are natural, healthy bodily processes and not in themselves diseases. On the other hand, he comments, "Pregnancy . . . may be considered as a strictly physiological state, but as one *bordering so closely upon the pathological*, that it is sometimes difficult to point out the boundary between them; and not infrequently this boundary is palpably transgressed."[72] And Dr. M. F. Billout comments, "Pregnancy, being a natural function, would seem to fall outside of the domain of the physician; but if we glance at what happens to the organization of the woman during this time, we will easily see the extremely sensitive state into which she is thrown, during which she finds herself exposed to a multitude of influences ["*impressions*"] that trouble her system."[73]

In the late modern imaginary, actual maternal bodies are neither stably fetishized nor written off as unruly. Rather, they perennially inhabit a slippery borderland between the two. From a bodily point of view, maternity is natural *at the border* of the pathological, threatening to 'transgress' into pathology at a moment's notice. The natural body of the Fetish Mother always expresses the 'essence' of maternality, while the hysterical body of the Unruly Mother always threatens to take over, and the boundary between these is difficult to discern and to patrol. Mothers' wombs and breasts are *essentially* or *naturally* perfect spaces that will generate order *if* they sustain a mythic level of perfect purity. But in fact, mundane bodies are messy and unpredictable in just the way that fetishized nature is not, and real mothers always harbor the potential to split from a unified whole into hysterical fragments. Thus actual mothers' bodies, in the wake of the Revolution, were subject to the interplay of distinct yet complementary pressures. They were glorified as spectacles and symbols of the natural order and *for the same reasons* policed as deeply untrustworthy and potentially unruly. Actual bodies were measured by the normative standards set by the Fetish Mother and at the same time governed by the anxieties surrounding the Unruly Mother. In the texts of the late eighteenth and nineteenth centuries, fetishistic glorifications of the maternal body are regularly juxtaposed with immediate warnings that real bodies can fall short at any moment. Real mothers' bodies thus became loci of ideological and practical stress and conflict. Insofar as they continuously fell short of incarnating the immaculate Fetish Mother and threatened unruliness and pathology, they revealed the insecurity that attended giving these bodies the responsibility for remaking second nature in the image of first nature.

Nowhere do we see this dynamic more clearly than in the domain of infant feeding, which from Rousseau onward has served as the privileged paradigm of a maternal bodily practice laden with formative powers and moral and political import. In the post-Rousseauian imagination, the *primary* power of the Fetish Mother is her capacity to well-order her children by keeping them proximate to her breast and bonded to her via milk. The nineteenth century witnessed a solidification of the Rousseauian notion that maternal breastfeeding is proper, natural, and a moral and social duty of mothers. Textbooks and guidebooks on infant rearing promoted breastfeeding not only through its health benefits but also by appealing to a normative notion of the natural order, and in particular the natural 'fit' between maternal breast and child. Coles writes, "the child was *made for* the breast and the breast was *made for* the child."[74] And according to Sebastian Kneipp, "No one goes unpunished who . . . leaves unfulfilled a Law of Nature. I warn every Mother who omits to fulfill the natural law written by God that she will not escape punishment which unhappily will fall also on her Child. Very many illnesses owe their origin to the evasion of the Law of Nature set down for the nourishment of the baby by the Mother itself."[75]

By the early twentieth century, with the professionalization of nursing, infant feeding along with the rest of infant care had been enshrined as a 'science': "The proper care of the baby consists in applying certain scientific health principles which have been reduced to working rules by specialists and made available for all mothers."[76] By this time, our basic current understanding of the nature and benefits of breast milk was already in place. Texts of the era outlined the character and benefits of colostrum, the mechanisms of milk production, the major health benefits of breastfeeding, and advice about appropriate schedules for weaning and feeding, much as our current texts do. This scientific turn brought with it a new interest in quantifying and monitoring the breastfeeding process. The Nazi state, which explicitly followed Rousseau in attributing to mothers' feeding practices the power to well-order or deform the citizenry, required Aryan mothers not only to nurse their children but also to have the volume of their milk production carefully measured, in order to ensure that they were not secretly letting their milk dry up.[77] Despite the new scientific and regulatory turn in infant feeding discourse and practices, the idea that breastfeeding was 'naturally' superior and that the breast and baby were 'meant for each other' remained intact.

But an integral part of the social fetishization of the 'natural' maternal body is the accompanying host of anxieties that its actual incarnation may be (and may have already been, without detection) violated and corrupted and transformed into an unruly body with porous boundaries that will spread deformity. Even while breastfeeding was enshrined as the ideal feeding method that expressed and incarnated proper, natural maternality, the nineteenth century saw the fermentation of a concern that particular mothers might be unsuited to breastfeeding—that their milk might be disordered, polluted, insufficient, or faulty for any of a number of reasons. Often within a single passage, we find the dual message that the maternal breast is the right, proper, natural source of nourishment *and* that actual breasts may be corrupted, treacherous, or deficient.[78]Even Rousseau himself could not trust actual maternal bodies with the very task he assigned to them in their fetishized form. He began *Emile*, as we know, with an impassioned lecture on the critical importance and healing powers of the maternal body, but then immediately and rather ironically removes Emile from his mother's care and places him in the hands of a wet nurse and a male tutor.[79] Mother's milk is apparently not always best after all. Like the courtesan's monstrous nipple, the maternal breast can betray its natural essence.

Alfred Donné, the discoverer of platelets and father of other crucial medical advances, affirms the normative status of maternal breastfeeding amidst an extraordinary litany of caveats:

If, then, there does not exist, either in the family of the mother or in her own person, any cutaneous or scrofulous affection, if no disposition to consumption is to be feared, if the temperament is not exceedingly lymphatic, if there is no tendency to any chronic disease, and if the mother is of ordinary strength and plumpness, if the appetite and the digestive functions are in good condition, if the strength is properly restored by food and sleep, and the milk is of good quality, and in sufficient quantity, nursing by the mother should not only be allowed, but it ought to be advised and encouraged.[80]

Mothers' milk could be 'spoiled' or 'disordered' by any number of compromising conditions, including, it will by now be no surprise, wayward and unregulated passions; "nothing disorders the milk so much as passion," Chavasse claims.[81] He prescribed artificial feeding methods to mothers of "weak constitution."[82] In turn, weak constitutions and bad temperaments in children were sometimes taken as *evidence* for poor-quality maternal milk due to an unruly maternal body,[83] which made for a rather unfalsifiable proposed causal connection.

Doctors could no longer trust the vague semiotic of the infant's body to reveal the quality of a mother's constitution after the fact. As we have seen, it was by now a matter of great civic importance to be able to tell which maternal bodies would produce order and which would produce disorder and monstrosity. Despite the grotesque images used to depict female wantonness and disorder in art, no one was confident that maternal depravity would be obvious to the naked or untrained eye. Thus a major medical project in the nineteenth century (significantly coincident with other characterological medical movements such as phrenology) was the search for principles for detecting and distinguishing between orderly and disorderly maternal bodies. As Fowler put it, we needed to know the "signs" for recognizing a "true woman" suited to bearing and nursing children—one with the proper "maternal qualifications."[84] The distinguished Dr. Donné took to examining mothers' milk under a microscope in order to determine its 'character,' so that he could develop a scientific system for determining which mothers should nurse their own children.[85] Thomas Bull devotes a chapter to the *detection* of "mothers who ought never to suckle," in which he catalogues various kinds of failed maternal bodies, including those with consumptive constitutions, those who are "nervous" or "precocious," and "the mother who only nurses her infant when it suits her convenience" instead of according to nature's calls.[86]

As the wet-nursing business declined and the artificial food industry began to develop seriously in the late nineteenth century, this double myth of the ideal breast and its disorderly instantiations shaped the evolving discourse and practices surrounding infant feeding. Formula feeding came to be increasingly recommended as an alternative for women with such deficient maternal bodies. Crucially, formula feeding was never promoted as an *improvement* upon normal maternal breastfeeding, and indeed maternal breastfeeding remained the official ideal with which infant formulas were compared. Maternal breasts may be best replaced, in certain cases, with scientifically engineered, publicly tested substitutes, but only when they had come under suspicion of unruliness and departure from the fetishized 'natural' breast. Infant formula manufacturers sought to broaden their market, *not* through the rhetoric of replacing nature with superior science, but rather through working to effect a proliferation of the ways in which maternal bodies could be special 'problem cases' for which their product was suitable.

It is no surprise that the artificial food industry found reasons to encourage some mothers to substitute their products for breast milk. What is interesting, for my purposes, about this early marketing is rather how 'pure' breast milk was presumed to be the ideal infant food even in the rhetoric of the formula manufacturers, who promoted their products as *closely simulating* proper maternal milk and as being the best substitute for mothers whose bodies and breasts had *failed* to remain pure and proper. According to one representative advertising pamphlet published by the Carnrick Company in 1890, "If you *find it necessary* to feed your child artificially, you certainly wish to give it the best Food and the one which is *most like human milk.* As milk is the food *provided by nature* for infants, it is certainly the only suitable material from which to manufacture an artificial food for young infants. The only Infant Foods ever prepared that *approach closely to human milk* in composition, digestibility and taste, are CARNRICK'S LACTO-PREPARATA AND CARNRICK'S SOLUBLE FOOD!"

The rhetoric surrounding infant feeding thus serves as a nice example of the twin, mutually constitutive normative pictures that between them shaped nineteenth-century attitudes toward actual mothers' bodies—bodies that did not wholly incarnate either the figure of the Fetish Mother or that of the Unruly Mother. On the one hand, the pure body of the Fetish Mother set up a standard for proper maternality, toward which mothers were expected to aspire. A proper mother would need no external interventions to raise her child in an orderly fashion, for her body would do so "naturally." On the other hand, mothers were warned of a plethora of ways in which their bodies could in fact fall short of this tribunal at a moment's notice and thereby require external regulation, surveillance, and aid. The ways in which these failings of the body could supposedly happen were so numerous and so mundane that it would be almost impossible to confidently control for all of them. Thus a culture of fetishistic faith in the powers of the ideal maternal body was pervaded with tropes and practices that undermined particular women's confidence in the trustworthiness of their own bodies.

———o———

In the first part of this book, I have explored what I take to have been a major conceptual, practical, ideological, scientific, and aesthetic shift in the status of mother's bodies—a shift that took shape in post-Rousseauian Revolutionary France and spread through Europe and to North America in the ensuing century. Out of this revolution, I have argued, emerged two mutually dependent yet in many ways opposite figurations of the maternal body that, separately and in interaction with one another, provided a complex lens through which actual mothers' bodies were interpreted and subjected to norms. Through these two maternal figures, the *space* and *boundaries* of mothers' bodies became contested sites, and our practical and imaginative understanding of proper and improper, natural and unnatural, appropriate and monstrous maternality came to be interpreted in spatial terms, such as unity, division, penetration, proximity, permeability, and displacement. Insofar as hysteria is distinctively a disorder and fragmentation grounded in a disordering of the space of the female reproductive body, we can read the late modern anxieties surrounding both maternal bodies themselves, and their impact upon the larger body politic, as hysterical anxieties. Concerns with the protection, penetration, and demarcation of the space of mothers' bodies shaped the norms that governed maternal practice and the care these bodies received. In the second half of this book, I pick up the contemporary narratives of the Unruly Mother and the Fetish Mother, and of the actual mothers' bodies that care and receive care through the complex interpretive and normative lenses these two figures provide. Despite major changes in the technological and social context in which mothers' bodies are situated, we will see that the basic form of these two maternal figures, their interaction, and their constitutive influence upon actual bodies and practices have remained reasonably constant. Our basic grasp of the maternal body is neither timeless nor new, but rather a distinctive development of the late Enlightenment era.

NOTES

1. William Buchan, *Advice to Mothers on the Subject of Their Own Health, and of the Means of Promoting the Health, Strength and Beauty of Their Offspring* (Boston: J. Bumstead, 1809), 1.

2. Several books have taken up this modern politicization of motherhood by way of a link between the work of mothers' bodies and the health of nations. Like me, Landes (2001) and Blum (1986) argue that this politicization is rooted in post-Rousseauian Revolutionary France. Oakley (1984) traces the nineteenth- and twentieth-century history of this nationalization of the maternal body. See Joan Landes, *Visualizing the Nation: Gender, Representation and Revolution in Eighteenth Century France* (Ithaca: Cornell University Press); Carol Blum, *Rousseau and the Republic of Virtue* (Ithaca: Cornell University Press, 1986); and Annie Oakley, *The Captured Womb: A History of the Medical Care of Pregnant Women* (London: Blackwell, 1984).

3. John Abbott, *The Mother at Home, or the Principles of Maternal Duty* (Boston: Crocker and Brewster, 1833), 147.

4. Michele Boulos Walker, *Philosophy and the Maternal Body: Reading Silence* (New York: Routledge, 1998), 138.

5. Landes 2001, 82. See her extended discussion and collection of these female grotesques in this work.

6. Landes 2001, 5.

7. "A tous les époques de sa vie, la femme inspire assurément le plus vif interêt: mais ne presenté-t-elle pas un tableau plus touchant encore lorsque, reçelant dans son sein la gage d'un amour sacré, elle assure un heritier à sa famille, un citoyen à la patrie! Quelle circonstance de la vie merité davantage, non-seulement l'attention du medicine, mais aussi du politique et du philosophe!" Billout, *Dissertation sur l'Hygiene des Femmes Encients* (Paris: Didot Jeune, 1816), 1, my translation and emphasis.

8. Barbara Duden, *Disembodying Women: Perspectives on Pregnancy and the Unborn*, trans. L. Hoinacki (Cambridge: Harvard University Press, 1993), 95.

9. See chapter 1.

10. Rousseau, *Emile, or On Education*, trans. A. Bloom (New York: Basic Books, 1979), 41.

11. *Emile*, 37.

12. *Emile*, 41, my emphasis.

13. *Emile*, 37, my emphasis.

14. Of course, our most famous monster, created by Dr. Frankenstein, has just this character. See the section Dissecting Monsters later in the chapter.

15. *Emile*, 37.

16. Jeremy Bentham, *The Panopticon Writings*, ed. M. Bozovic (New York: Verso, 1995). Bentham's Panopticon has been made most familiar through Michel Foucault's discussion of it in *Discipline and Punish: The Birth of the Prison* (New York: Pantheon, 1977).

17. O. S. Fowler, *Maternity: Or the Bearing and Nursing of Children, Including Female Education and Beauty* (New York: Fowler and Wells, 1856), 15–16.

18. Fowler 1856, 17.

19. P. H. Chavasse, *The Physical Training of Children* (Philadelphia: New World Publishing Co., 1872), 19 and throughout.

20. Hopkinson, *Hints for the Nursery, or the Young Mother's Guide* (Boston: Little, Brown and Co., 1863), 11–12.

21. Duden, *The Woman Beneath the Skin* (Cambridge: Harvard University Press, 1991), 17.

22. Like other new techniques that involved touching or penetrating the maternal body, such as dissections and even stethoscope use, palpation was first used only on unmarried pregnant women.

23. Quoted at Duden 1993, 96.

24. See for instance Walter Coles, *The Nurse and Mother: A Manual for the Guidance of Monthly Nurses and Mothers* (Chicago: J. H. Chambers and Co., 1881).

25. Hopkinson 1863, 14, 29. Indeed, by 1932, the physician's eye had become an irreplaceable measure of maternal function and an element of responsible prenatal practice in and of itself: "No matter how much a mother knows, whether she is a doctor, a nurse, a midwife, or a mother who has other children, there is only one way that she can ever be *sure* that her body is doing its best work. That is to be examined by a good doctor as soon as she thinks she might be pregnant and to follow his advice." The Maternity Center Association of New York, *Maternity Handbook for Pregnant Mothers and Expectant Fathers* (New York: Putnam and Sons, 1932), 15.

26. See M. Foucault, *The Birth of the Clinic: An Archaeology of Medical Perception* (New York: Vintage Books, 1984). The quotation is from xii.

27. See for instance S. Farr, *Elements Of Medical Jurisprudence; Or A Succinct And Compendious Description Of Such Tokens In The Human Body As Are Requisite To Determine The Judgment Of A Coroner, And Courts Of Law, In Cases Of Divorce, Rape, Murder &C. To Which Are Added, Directions For Preserving The Public Health* (London: Callow, 1815).

28. Foucault 1984, 34.

29. Foucault 1984, 34.

30. Foucault 1984, 19.

31. Quoted at Foucault 1984, 146.

32. Cited in T. Bull, *Hints to Mothers, for the Management of Health During the Period of Pregnancy, and in the Lying-In Room* (New York: J. Wiley, 1842), 20.

33. Hunter, *Anatomy of the Human Gravid Uterus* (Birmingham: J. Baskerville, 1774), preface, my emphasis.

34. Hunter 1774, caption to Plate VI.

35. Some prominent examples, in addition to Smellie's text, include James Blundell, *The Principles and Practice of Obstetrics as at Present Taught* (Washington: Duff Green, 1834); Samuel Bard, *A Compendium of the Theory and Practice of Midwifery* (New York: Collins and Co., 1817); James Burns, *Principles of Midwifery* (New York: Joseph H. Francis, 1837); P. Cazeaux, *A Theoretical and Practical Treatise on Midwifery, Including the Diseases of Pregnancy and Parturition*, trans. R. P. Thomas (Philadelphia: Lindsay and Blakiston, 1805); and several widely read works by Fleetwood Churchill, including *On the Diseases of Women; Including Those of Pregnancy and Childbirth* (Philadelphia: Blanchard and Lea, 1857); and *On the Theory and Practice of Midwifery* (Philadelphia: Blanchard and Lea, 1860).

36. Smellie 1754, ix.

37. Examples of these texts include several I have already cited, such as Buchan 1809, Fowler 1856, Chavasse 1872, and Coles 1881. Other interesting examples include Father Sebastian Kneipp (the father of hydrotherapy!), *The Care of Children in Sickness and Health*, 1896 (Reprinted by Kenssinger Publisher, 2004); and John Abbott, *A Mother at Home* (Boston: Crocker and Brewster, 1833), which still has a cult following in conservative pro-natalist communities, such as the online community "Blessed Mother," and continues to be reprinted in paperback by Christian presses.

38. Kneipp 1896, 19.

39. Fowler 1856, 105.

40. Fowler 1856, 131.

41. Chavasse 1872, 44.

42. See for instance Buchan 1809.

43. Coles 1881, 128–29, 30, emphasis in the original.

44. Buchan 1809, 72ff., 75.

45. Buchan 1809, 33.

45. Buchan 1809, 33.

46. The notion of commodity fetishization has of course spawned a vast literature, but the classic original discussion and definition appears in Marx's *Economic and Philosophical Manuscripts of 1844* (New York: International Publishers, 1980).

47. See Slavoj Žižek, *The Sublime Object of Ideology* (New York: Verso, 1989), for one excellent discussion and analysis of the logic and ideological structure of fetishes. My account here is inspired by his but streamlined to suit my present needs.

48. Foucault 1984, 31.

49. Buchan 1809, 30.

50. Landes 2001, 21, 78.

51. This risk was seen as quite literal; remember that it was 'unnatural,' cosmopolitan women who thwarted the traditional narratives of wife and mother who were most often diagnosed as hysterics and seen as most at risk for the illness.

52. Churchill 1857, 447–48.

53. Bull 1842, 31–2.

54. Churchill 1857, 488–90.

55. See for example Churchill 1857; Buchan 1809; and J. C. Petit, *Woman: Her Physical Condition, Sufferings and Maternal Relations. A Course of Parlor Lectures to Ladies* (self-published, St. Louis, 1895).

56. Petit 1895, 30, 36.

57. Abbott 1833, 64.

58. Churchill 1857, 458–59.

59. John Blunt, *Man-Midwifery Dissected* (London: S. W. Fores, 1793); Philip Thicknesse, *Man-Midwifery Analyzed* (London: R. Davis, 1764); Samuel Gregory, *Man-Midwifery Exposed and Corrected* (Boston: G. Gregory, 1848). See also Elizabeth Nihell, *A Treatise on the Art of Midwifery, Setting Forth Various Abuses Therein, Especially as to the Practice with Instruments* (London: A. Morely, 1760); Anonymous, *An Important Address to Wives and Mothers on the Dangers and Immorality of Man-Midwifery* (London: Lewis and Co., 1830).

60. See the section "The Truth Was Thereby Well Authenticated." It was in England that the routine monitoring of pregnancy and birth was most quickly moving into professional male hands, and this was also the country housing the most vocal opponents of the shift (although, oddly, these critics generally blamed the French for the trend).

61. Blunt 1793, xii.

62. Blundell 1834, 142–43.

63. See for instance Blundell 1834 and Smellie 1754.

64. Thicknesse 1764, 2–3.

65. Blunt 1793, 165.

66. Smellie 1754, 241, my emphasis.

67. Shelley, preface to the 1831 edition of *Frankenstein*.

68. The literate and curious young Shelley would likely have been familiar with the debates surrounding man-midwifery, which got a fair amount of popular press at the time.

69. Wells, *The Island of Dr. Moreau*, ed. R. M. Philmus (Athens, GA: University of Georgia Press, 1896/1993), 50.

70. Wells 1896/1993, 51.

71. President Bush's National Bioethics Council, charged with being the state keepers of bioethical integrity in a nation riddled with racial disparities in health, millions of uninsured children, HIV, astronomical drug prices, a pharmaceutical lobby with almost unlimited power, crippling litigiousness, rising rates of morbid obesity, and an epidemic of asthma and developmental delays among poor children living in polluted ur-

ban centers, has devoted most of its time to expressing its imaginative discomfort with such fantasies of scientifically controlled, displaced reproduction. See www.bioethics .gov/reports/ for a list of their publications.

72. Churchill 1857, 441, my emphasis.

73. "La grossesse, étant une function naturelle, paraîtrait, par cela-même, hors du domaine de la medicine; mais si nous jetons un coup d'oeil sur ce qui se passé alors dans l'organization de la femme, nous verrons façilement que l'extreme sensibilité dont elle jouit, et l'état de suceptibilité dans lequelle elle se trouve à cette époque l'exposent à une multitude d'impressions qui jettent un trouble dans son economie." Billout 1816, 7, my translation.

74. Coles 1881, 143.

75. Kneipp 1896, 52–53.

76. U.S. Department of Labor Children's Bureau, *Infant Care* (Washington, DC: Government Printing Office, 1926), 11.

77. Miriam Yalom, *A Short History of the Breast* (New York: Ballantine Books, 1997), 140.

78. It is of course tempting to offer psychoanalytic explanations of these two images of the maternal breast. Many feminist theorists have devoted time to Freudian or Lacanian or object relations analyses of our social construal of our relation to the maternal body. Melanie Klein certainly offers a story that prefigures and could be seen as explaining my account of the two mother figures. On her account, the process of identity formation occurs through the relationship to the maternal breast, which is seen as double: the 'bad breast' is taken as a threat to the survival and independence of the infant self, while the 'ideal breast' is construed as endlessly satisfying and nurturing. (See Walker 1998 for a clear and sympathetic summary of Melanie Klein's variation on psychoanalytic doctrine.) I will not take up such explanations or assess their worth. It seems to me, though, that to the extent that we can sort out causal dependencies, psychoanalytic accounts have their roots in ideological and historical pressures, more than the reverse. In any case, my interest here is with this ideological genesis rather than with any psychological genesis that may or may not coincide with it.

79. In fact, the tutor so thoroughly supplants the mother that he takes over the natural proximity and absolute identity with his charge that ideally characterizes the mother-infant relationship, and then the citizen-*patrie* relationship, for Rousseau: "I would even want the pupil and the governor to regard themselves as so inseparable that the lot of each in life is always a common object for them. As soon as they envisage from afar their separation, as soon as they foresee the moment which is going to make them strangers to one another, they are already strangers" (*Emile*, 53).

80. Donné, *Mothers and Infants, Nurses and Nursing* (Boston: Phillips, Spapson and Co., trans. 1859), 39.

81. Chavasse 1872, 50.

82. Chavasse 1872, 26.

83. For instance see Coles 1881, 146.

84. Fowler 1856, 59.

85. Donné 1842.

86. Bull 1842, 196ff.

PART
2

4

The Uterus as Public Theater

The Unruly Mother, with her dangerously permeable boundaries and her insides capable of creating disorder and monstrosity, has survived and flourished over the last few centuries. So has the Fetish Mother, with her extended boundaries and her power to create normative natural order with her body. In part II of this book, I will try to give some of the contemporary biography of these two maternal bodies, as they are reinscribed within contemporary North American culture, and to explore how actual mothers' bodily practices and identity are constituted and measured by these two maternal figures.

My focus in this chapter will be on how *pregnant* bodies are figured as unruly, and my focus in the two following chapters will be on how the bodies of *new mothers* are fetishized, or held to standards set by the Fetish Mother. I do think—and I will try to show—that this division has some hegemony. That is, I think that (contemporary North American) maternal bodies are generally imagined as potentially unruly while they are pregnant and held to fetishized standards after they give birth. In my concluding chapter, I will discuss the significance of this ideological division of labor. But the division is a matter of emphasis. There are stories to be told about fetishizations of the pregnant body that gestates and gives birth without artificial, alien interruptions, and also about how newly maternal bodies are treated as inherently unruly and untrustworthy. Some of these stories will come out in chapters 6 and 7. We need to remember, as I pick out what I believe are dominant narratives in the next few chapters, that imaginings of maternal bodies as unruly and as fetishized are always two sides of the same ideological coin, and they always complement and constitute one another—I argued this at some length in chapter 3. However, I will tell a reasonably unified story here, in order to make a case for the ability of the bodies of the Unruly Mother and the Fetish Mother to function as concrete cultural forces constituting mothers' bodies and boundaries, without trying to give an exhaustive account of the complex ideological lives of maternal bodies.

SETTING THE STAGE

The logic of the maternal imagination, which turns pregnant women's skins into fully permeable media, ready to transmit directly to the fetus the substances that the pregnant woman ingests, still governs our cultural imagination.[1] We take the womb as a space that must be kept pure in order to perform its task of producing well-ordered nature, and we also take this space as easily corrupted from without, and thereby transformed into a dangerous laboratory of monstrosity. A 1985 book on the effect of environmental contaminants on fetuses is entitled *The Poison Womb: Human Reproduction in a Polluted World*;[2] here neither the world nor the fetus is rhetorically presented as poison, but only the womb itself. A 1973 work subtitled "Influences of the Prenatal Environment" begins, "This book represents an effort to catalogue forces in the maternally imposed environment that can penetrate the protective mechanisms available to the fetus and significantly alter the outcome of pregnancy."[3] In these cases, the pregnant woman shows up only insofar as she 'imposes' a toxic environment upon her fetus.

Our obsession with expectant mothers' temptations toward inappropriate, irrational ingestion has remained equally alive. If we look up *pregnancy* as a subject heading on a modern academic library catalogue, we find that over 80% of the primary subheadings concern women's corruptions of the insides of their own bodies, specifically through their inappropriate ingestions. These subheadings catalogue the substances that underdisciplined women with weak boundaries and strong appetites are at risk of inviting or allowing into the pure space of their wombs: alcohol, tobacco, crack, excessive amounts of food, unhealthy foods, environmental toxins, marijuana, and so forth. As in the premodern and modern eras, it is still women's cravings and passions, as well as the transparent openness of her womb to disordering influences, that are feared as the sources of deformed human nature.

In response to her own craven appetites and the permeability of her body, the proper pregnant woman is still expected to cultivate rigorous self-discipline and to police her boundaries and appetites. Markens, Browner, and Press point out that "from commercials and friends to warnings in restaurants and remarks by complete strangers,

U.S. pregnant women are constantly reminded that they need to manage and control themselves during pregnancy. The invariant message is that what they do, and to an even greater extent what they *consume*, can directly affect the fetus growing inside them."[4] As one prenatal instructor expressed it, "Anything you put in your mouth, anything you smoke, anything you snort up your nose will go to the baby."[5] Pregnancy guides tell women that every single bite they put in their mouths is (ethically and medically) important and that they should imagine each of these bites as being fed *directly* to the baby.[6] We are gripped by a kind of third-person anorexia when it comes to the disciplining of pregnant bodies—an anorexia that, as we saw, dates back at least 400 years.[7]

Our mass hysteria over the permeability of the mother's boundaries, along with her propensities toward ingestion, though no doubt incorporating large elements of medical fact, must be read as having a strong ideological and even mythic component to it, as this permeability is rhetorically exhibited, enforced, and exaggerated. A 1989 controlled study showed that papers supporting the negative effect of a drug on 'pregnancy outcome' were more likely to be accepted at scientific conferences than those demonstrating a negligible effect of a drug on outcome, even when the latter were better designed by standard methodological criteria.[8] Katha Pollit points out that "our basic model is 'innocent' fetuses that would be fine if only presumably 'guilty' mothers refrained from indulging in their 'whims,'" while other dramatic dangers to infants' health, such as poverty, racism, and male violence, are rhetorically eclipsed.[9] The widespread emphasis on maternal indulgence and ingestion has come at the cost of systematic attention to such other factors, which have provably larger effects on fetal outcome.[10]

In chapter 1, we saw that before the institutionalized medicalization of childbirth and prenatal care in the late eighteenth century, the inside of the female human body, and especially the pregnant body, was very poorly understood. In chapter 3, we saw how new pressures on maternal bodies to serve as seats of civic harmony and moral order converged with this institutionalized medicalization and with the corresponding quest to open up the space of the womb for public surveillance, examination, and scientific regulation. From the late eighteenth century onward, Duden writes, "step by step, the physician's finger, then his stethoscope, later x-rays, tests, and sonar have invaded woman's gendered interior and opened it to the non-gendered public gaze."[11] From a strictly visual point of view, the widespread use of ultrasound imaging and fetal monitoring during pregnancy and labor have publicized the space of the uterus, both by making its contents visually accessible, and more specifically by making them accessible literally elsewhere than at the site of the mother's body. Ultrasound technicians check the status of fetuses by looking at a screen, not at the mother. Nurses and doctors judge the progress of labor and make decisions about interventions by looking at readings on a fetal monitor, which serves as the gauge for the reality of the laboring woman's contractions. Some women feel oddly alienated during labor when they realize that health care workers literally and regularly turn *away* from them during a contraction so as to better see the monitor; some report feeling as if it is the machine that is having the baby, rather than them.[12] (My own very attentive and supportive husband and labor coach took to 'informing' me of when I was having a contraction, according to the monitor—a piece of redundant information bound to infuriate any laboring woman writhing in excruciating pain.) Thus the hysterical displacement of the uterus into public space had become visually literalized with the advent of new surveillance technologies. Indeed, many feminist bioethicists have pointed out that the current explosion of new and relatively accessible possibilities for fetal monitoring, testing and intervention have transformed prenatal care from care for pregnant women into an "interaction among the health provider, the woman, and the fetus."[13]

At the level of policy, the insides of the pregnant woman's body are coming to have an institutionalized public status quite distinct from that of the mother, and potentially in conflict with hers; no doubt the visual publicity of these insides helps to imaginatively support the acceptance of this status. Pregnant women have recently begun to be prosecuted for using drugs during pregnancy, on the grounds of their wrongfully endangering the life of a child. In the United States, laws enacted in the last few years have made fetal homicide a separate crime and have instituted separate protections for fetal participants in 'human' subjects research. George W. Bush has recently proposed granting fetuses their own separate health insurance under SCHIP, a state-run medical insurance plan for low-income children.[14] This program would grant separate recognition and protection to a part of a woman's body independently of the rest of it, perhaps without her even being in a position to purchase the same recognition and protection for herself. The possibility that a better-protected fetus may be 'entitled' to medical procedures at the direct expense of the mother's health, without her being able to afford counterprotection, immediately looms. Such policies and programs do not adjudicate between conflicting rights but rather help constitute or concretize the fetus as a possible rights-bearer located in civic space.

We saw that this move toward fetal publicity had its roots in the late Enlightenment. Its current intensification is a product of new technologies in combination with political pressures that intensify rather than revise our grasp of the boundaries of maternal bodies. A growing number of feminist scholars have demonstrated and discussed the new publicity of the uterus and have argued that this publicity has helped to grant imaginative and political personhood to fetuses.[15] While I am in sympathy with these discussions and appreciate the readings of contemporary culture they proffer, I do think that these critiques have tended to be problematically ahistorical. Although many of our techniques for fetal surveillance are new, I hope to have already shown that our urge to convert the maternal body into a public space and to put the fetus on public display has time-honored, deeply modernist roots. Since the eighteenth century, our valuing of the fetus as socially precious and our desire to protect it from its untrustworthy 'maternal environment' have expressed themselves in a progressive, Benthamite transformation of the space of the maternal body into a public arena. We hysterically displace the uterus and fetus into public space in order to cure and prevent the hysteria that can be spread from the unruly maternal body.

On the other hand, I do think that new developments in the material and rhetorical context and practices surrounding contemporary North American pregnancy have altered what we might think of as the ontology of pregnancy, including the ontology of fetuses and pregnant maternal bodies. Hence my story here is one of both continuity and discontinuity. My specific argument will be that contemporary technologies and rituals (in contrast to their eighteenth- and nineteenth-century counterparts) have produced a *single*, canonical fetus who has become the inhabitant of each individual pregnant body, as well as a *shared*, public pregnancy narrative that constitutes and interprets each individual pregnancy. In the course of these productions, women's own construal of the configuration of their bodies and boundaries, and of their relationship to the fetuses and children that inhabit these bodies and confound these boundaries, has been profoundly changed. I will try to show how the womb has become a public, rigorously regulated space and how pregnant women use a set of public rituals and images to forge and personalize a mediated, third-person relationship with the contents of their own displaced, shared insides.

The publicity of the fetus, and the ethical and ontological significance of this publicity with respect to the negotiation of the boundaries of maternal bodies, has mainly been discussed by recent scholars in two contexts: one is analyses of the abortion debate, and the other

is discussions of prenatal testing and fetal surveillance that are primarily concerned with cases in which a fetal abnormality or future disability is detected.[16] Both sets of scholars are concerned with how this
fetal publicity can set up a problematically antagonistic relationship
between a pregnant woman and her fetus. I have found both of these
bodies of literature to be important, largely convincing, and indeed a
major inspiration for my own work. However, I think the extent to
which these discourses have focused on the relatively exceptional
cases of 'problematic' pregnancies—problematic because of the position of either the fetus or the mother—is highly significant. We have
spent vastly less theoretical time analyzing the impact of these same
rituals and practices on 'normal' pregnancies, in which the fetus appears to be healthy and the mother has already made or simply presumed the decision to bring the pregnancy to term and keep the child.
I am not suggesting that this notion of normalcy does not require critical and normative interrogation. However, *most* pregnancies are
healthy and accepted, and something very strange and problematic
happens to our critical and theoretical stance when we focus our analytic attention almost entirely on the minority of cases where the 'normal' narrative *goes wrong*. To do so is not only to get a biased picture
of the social reality of pregnancy but also to implicitly presume that
healthy, accepted, normal pregnancies are somehow immune from the
constitutive power of rhetoric, ideology, and politics and unmarked by
social practices and meanings, or that they form an innocent or 'natural' terrain where no ethical and rhetorical interrogation is required.
Almost no contemporary theorists would explicitly accept such pre-
sumptions, and yet most books and articles that discuss the constitution of fetal and maternal bodies and their relations to one another
cast their entire discussions in terms that begin with the politics of
what we might call 'exceptional' pregnancies.[17] My aim here, then, is
to take the less traveled path and to attend first and foremost to the
rhetorical and ideological structure and ritual practices that constitute
such normal, healthy, embraced pregnancies.

THE 'SONOGRAPHIC VOYEUR'
AND THE RITUALS OF FETAL RECOGNITION

In *Disembodying Women: Perspectives on Pregnancy and the Unborn*, historian Barbara Duden writes,

> Now we are overwhelmed with fetuses. I encountered one recently in
> a German ad for a Swedish car. Another one confronted me from the

top of a circular urging me to discuss abortion with my candidate before giving him my vote. . . . How did the unborn turn into a billboard image and how did that isolated goblin get into the limelight? How did the female peritoneum acquire transparency?[18]

Some members of the medical community have not been shy in their rhetoric when it comes to the project of turning the uterus into a public theater and the fetus into its lead actor. A 1981 article in the *Journal of the American Medical Association* announced that:

> The fetus could not be taken seriously [the authors do not say by whom] as long as he remained a medical recluse in an opaque womb; and it was not until the last half of this century that the prying eye of the ultrasonogram . . . rendered the once opaque womb transparent, stripping the veil of mystery from the dark inner sanctum and letting the light of scientific observation fall upon the shy and secretive fetus. . . . The sonographic voyeur, spying on the unwary fetus, finds him or her a surprisingly active little creature, and not at all the passive parasite that we [again, it is not specified who] had imagined.[19]

One feature that distinguishes the fetus who is coaxed out of the opaque womb and shows up on the German billboard from its eighteenth-century counterparts is its *singularity*. The fetus is here represented as a *character* who can be found in various wombs and public spaces, starring in movies such as *2001: A Space Odyssey*, and picking up advertising endorsements. The insides of the pregnant body have been transformed into a theatrical public space, and the fetus has correspondingly become a kind of public celebrity. The fetus that has come into view in the brightly lit arena of the scientific and public gaze has a recognizable visual identity, which is familiar to us by way of everything from anti-abortion propaganda to public health pamphlets for pregnant women to science fiction movies and science shows for kids. While the medical and social institutions of the eighteenth century tentatively strove to make public the spaces of particular women's bodies and the fetuses they contained, this *common*, shared fetus with its familiar look and its distinctive personality has been enabled—as we shall see—by much more recent politics and technology.

The official position of the fetus, with respect to the viewer, is curled up with its side facing us—in other words, in the fetal position, although any pregnant woman who has made it into her fifth month will have a hard time believing that there is such a thing as 'the' position of a being whose limbs can clearly be felt flailing in all directions. The skin of the official fetus is pink, and it emits a soft glow against a dark background. The umbilical cord trails off into nothingness, leaving the fetus to present itself as a self-subsistent entity. A specific photographer, Lennart Nilsson, together with the editors of *Life* magazine, in fact engineered this look for the human fetus. Nilsson was a pioneer in techniques of endoscopic fetal imaging. His work was made public with much fanfare in a 1965 issue of *Life*, after his having worked closely with the editors of the magazine over a twelve-year period, and his images were further canonized in the influential book *A Child Is Born*, its iconic cover showing a silhouette of a pregnant torso, whose glowing, transparent belly reveals the head of an enormous fetus in the fetal position sucking its thumb.[20] The technology Nilsson used forced him and his editors to confront substantial choice points with respect to how his final images would look. Not surprisingly, they chose in the directions that maximized how attractive, sympathetic, and human the fetus looked. The official status of this visual identity is repeatedly and ritualistically reinforced in various ways. For instance, ultrasound technicians, who examine fetuses from all sorts of undignified perspectives, invariably choose an image of the fetus that mimics Nilsson's representational conventions to turn into a snapshot for parents to keep.

As Barbara Duden puts it, Nilsson's images have become "part of the mental universe of our time."[21] But most pertinent, for my purposes, is the extent to which such images have co-opted *pregnant women's* imaginations—that is, the extent to which many pregnant women can accept Nilsson's glowing creature as a representation of the inhabitant of their own bodies. The power of these public representations of the fetus over our imaginations and self-understandings during pregnancy is not simply a product of their being so widespread. Rather, their effective co-option of the pregnant imagination has much to do with how many pregnant women have come to have a third-person relationship to their own insides. Expectant mothers' own relationships to the insides of their bodies is powerfully mediated by public measures and representations. We have no visual access to our fetuses other than through public representations, and our tactile access, which used to be the main measure of the reality and status of the fetus, has been dwarfed by robust public representations and their imaginative power.[22]

I want to argue that women understand their own pregnancies in and through an elaborate set of public measures and inscriptions that together construct a single, canonical public pregnancy and a canonical, fungible, shared fetus with a scientifically surveyable and quantifiable identity.[23] Forging an individualized bond with this public figure, I claim, has become a special kind of project for the pregnant woman—one that is understood to be an important part of a conscientious pregnancy. Contemporary technologies, and the rhetorical and ideological context in which they are used, encourage us each to think of *our* fetus—the one to which we are expected to feel a unique bond and responsibility—through the medium of and with reference to generic public representations.

Ritualized events such as hearing the fetus' amplified heartbeat for the first time and receiving a keepsake ultrasound snapshot are effectively socially constituted as crucial moments of bonding. These are rituals that are shared with others—usually at least the other parent and a health provider. Women are encouraged to treat the shared character of these events as part of their emotional portent, as is clear in one current television commercial for new, increasingly 'lifelike' 3-D ultrasound imaging, which shows a heterosexual couple holding hands and crying as they see their 'baby' on the screen for the first time. Eugenia Georges and Lisa Mitchell found that Canadian ultrasound technicians regularly encourage or even demand that fathers actively participate in this event of 'seeing the baby.'[24] Furthermore, these milestones occur at ritualized times during the pregnancy: usually the twelfth week for the heartbeat and the nineteenth week for the ultrasound. Thus they help bring the pregnancies themselves, along with their 'personalized' moments of 'bonding,' under a common narrative and timetable. Significantly, these two milestones are often chosen by expectant parents as the moments that mark when it is 'safe' to 'make the pregnancy public' and hence to begin the process of giving it concrete social and institutional reality as an authentic pregnancy.

Indeed, women routinely take the 'successful' ultrasound as a definitive marker of the 'reality' of the fetus. Lisa Mitchell, in her study of pregnant Canadian women of very diverse racial, class, and linguistic backgrounds, found that three-quarters of the women described their babies and their pregnancies as gaining some kind of new, enhanced reality through the nineteenth-week ultrasound screening.[25] Lorna Weir makes the same point in the context of her similar study of American women, and she also found that 'keepsake' ultrasound photos were often used to make pregnancy announcements; thus the ultrasound image literally served as an introduction of the fetus into the public sphere.[26] It is these shared milestones, rather than old-fashioned internally available moments such as quickening, that we now take as critical moments for the establishment of the fetus as a 'real baby' with public status and as an individualized object of our care and affection.[27]

Mitchell and Georges[28] documented how Canadian ultrasound technicians enact rituals that help the images serve as devices for 'personalizing' parents' relationship to their fetus. Avoiding the use of the word *fetus*, the technicians routinely talk informally to the parents about what the 'baby' on the screen is thinking and feeling, and during the ultrasound they talk *to* the fetus in ways that playfully presume its independent and individualized agency—for instance, by accusing it of being 'shy' or 'modest' when its genitals prove hard to see.[29] But at the same time, alongside these personalizing rituals, the ultrasound technicians are uncomfortable with and even verbally judgmental toward prospective parents who seemed very interested in knowing their baby's sex, telling them that "finding out the sex isn't important. The most important thing is that the baby is healthy"; sometimes, especially in the case of nonwhite patients, the technicians simply lied about being able to discern the sex of the fetus.[30] Thus the technicians' discourse pushes in both the directions I am tracing: they use the images that they control in order to help canonize an image of a fungible public fetus, unindividuated even by sex, and they also facilitate the forging of a personalized relationship with this fetus by presenting it to its parents as a humanized interlocutor.

After a routine ultrasound, Mitchell found, women regularly adopt the language of their sonographer as their own. That is, women often report what the *sonographer* said that *she* saw as what *they* saw, using the same terms as the sonographer used. This phenomenon is an interesting marker of the extent to which expectant mothers' relationships to their fetuses is third-personal and mediated by public representations. Ultrasound images themselves are notoriously hard to read, and only a trained eye can make much of them. But women report that they 'saw' that the baby's femur was of a certain size, indicating a certain gestational age, and so forth.[31] They thus adopt the mediating third-person stance of the sonographer as their own for the purposes of understanding their encounter with their fetuses through the ultrasound image.

Routine ultrasounds play a social rather than a narrowly medical purpose.[32] Empirical study has yielded no significant medical benefits to routine ultrasound screening, with respect to any fetal or maternal outcomes, including maternal anxiety. Despite these results, ultrasound screening has been increasingly and dramatically routinized, and it is regularly covered by health insurance plans. For women whose voracious ultrasound needs are not being satiated in the setting of traditional prenatal care, ultrasound booths have now set up shop in upscale malls, and employees will show women their babies and give them a keepsake photo for a fee. Franchises such as Peek A Boo Baby do not offer their technicians trainings in how to detect fetal abnormalities or break bad news; the presumption governing these booths is that the fetus is healthy and that the service they offer is not a med-

ical service at all, but rather that of 'introducing' expectant mothers to
their babies and providing them with keepsake photos and videos (see
figure 4.1).[33] The technological ritual of fetal ultrasound is thus perceived by the health industry, the private sector, and pregnant women
alike as meeting some important need, and this need is not medical.
Ultrasounds have come to play an important role in what we understand as the *appropriate* epistemics of pregnancy and the formation of
appropriate maternal-fetal relations. In the majority of cases, the procedures function (and are understood by women) first and foremost as
social rituals of personification, normalization, displacement, and
bonding rather than as diagnostic procedures.[34]

Scholars of 'prenatal diagnosis' who have focused on cases where
tests show an 'abnormal' fetus, such as Barbara Katz Rothman and Rayna
Rapp, have powerfully portrayed how routinized prenatal testing makes
pregnancies importantly 'tentative' (to use Rothman's influential term)
until the tests come back negative, and how this changes the ethical contours and experience of pregnancy. Against this background, they argue
that the choice to undergo prenatal testing has complicated moral significance, independent of what choices we might make about continuing a
pregnancy in the face of the test results (although obviously these choices
are also morally weighty and complicated).

But by focusing on cases where pregnant women receive abnormal
results from tests, such scholars risk importantly skewing the normal
ethical structure of these rituals of prenatal testing. Both anthropolog-
ical studies[35] and common sense suggest that most women, as long as
they are not already at high risk for some specific reason, and despite
a generally manageable dose of pregnancy anxiety, (quite rationally)

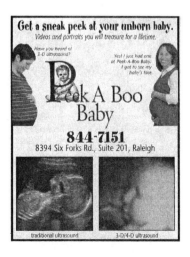

Figure 4.1. "Peek A Boo Baby," advertisement, 2003.

expect that the routine prenatal tests that they undergo will help affirm the health of their babies. Thus their decision to undergo the procedures does not actually function, for them, as an act of putting the
fetus itself to the test (although if the tests show a problem, this understanding will have to be revised in situ).[36] Indeed, although the critical literature tends to talk about prenatal 'diagnosis,' these tests function socially as *diagnostic* only when they turn up an abnormality. In
most cases, ultrasounds and other routine tests serve to affirm and to
grant legitimacy to a pregnancy that was never really in question. The
'tests,' in the normal cases, function socially much more as rituals of
concretization, bonding, and publicization than they function as dramatic ethical choice points.

Furthermore, it is not even clear that women generally make ethically discrete *decisions* to undergo testing in the first place. Many prenatal tests such as ultrasounds are now so routinized that there is not
actually an identifiable moment at which a woman *chooses* to undergo them; normally, doctors simply take it as a matter of course that
women will have these tests and women simply follow their doctors'
recommendations.[37]Lisa Mitchell points out that no maternal consent
is required for ultrasound screenings. But even in the case of tests that
do require consent, such as amniocenteses and maternal blood screening tests, we should by no means assume that the *formal* moment of
consent is interpreted (by the woman or by her health providers) as an
important and well-defined moment of choice with ethical weight.[38]
Often, signing the consent form is *itself* routinized as part of normal
prenatal care, and the 'choice' to undergo the test reveals itself as a
moral crossroads only in retrospect, if a positive result throws the status of the pregnancy into sharp relief.

It is important to pay attention to the fact that the results of routinized fetal surveillance, particularly fetal heartbeats and mid-
pregnancy ultrasounds, all sound and look more or less identical, as
long as the fetus is healthy. Notice that the ultrasound photos in figure 4.1 are treated as exemplary: they advertise the images that *each
customer* will receive. Thus our pleasure in these first 'encounters'
with our 'baby' is inextricably bound up with our pleasure in the con-
formation of our experience to the shared norm. It is to some extent
the very normalcy of our fetus—its instantiation of a single, homoge-
neous fetal form—that serves to socially entrench its reality and to establish our personal bond with it. This point is strikingly underlined
by the fact that, as Weir documents, women whose ultrasounds detect
a fetal abnormality are *not* provided with the keepsake photos that
their counterparts receive.[39] This means that everyone who is participating in the rituals of personification that make up normal ultra-

sound practice ends up personifying more or less the *same* image, and one that has been stamped as conforming to the norm. We have paid a lot of critical attention to how the fetus is 'personified' in the context of the rhetoric and representations around pregnancy, with potent consequences for the politics of abortion. But we need to notice that this personification process is not simply an *individualization* process. On the contrary, the rituals of pregnancy importantly serve to homogenize and normalize the pregnant narrative and the fetal object.

The various pregnancy 'tools' that are now available on the Internet are excellent examples of technologies that help produce and authenticate both generic representations of the fetus—streamlined pregnancy experiences—and our individualized, attached relationship to the fetus through them. Their advertisements tell pregnant women that "you can see what *your baby* looks like *right now*" or that "you can track *your baby's* growth and development." The way these tools generally work is that 'you' enter your due date into a program that will then produce a series of descriptions of 'your' child based on this information. Often, evolving descriptions and images are e-mailed to 'your' personal account on a weekly basis. Other programs produce a 'personalized' calendar with daily descriptions of changes in 'your baby,' such as 'your baby now enjoys sucking her thumb,' or 'your baby can now recognize your voice.' At www.babycenter.com, you can now subscribe, for $12, to a service that will e-mail you weekly videos offering "personalized updates on the stages of your pregnancy."[40] Like the sonographers' discourse, these tools do double work: they use generic information to construct a canonical public fetus and to entrench the idea that this common fetus *is* what is inside *your* body, while at the same time they rhetorically constitute a personalized relationship with this public figure.

It is perhaps ironic but nearly inevitable that such tools, by presenting us with representations and information that are completely fungible, will make the fetus within us feel like more of an 'individual' with whom we can bond. Georges and Mitchell found that many women describe themselves as reading public literature about pregnancy as a way of 'getting involved' in their own pregnancies.[41] It is interesting to notice, here, how pregnant women have come to take it as an important goal in the first place that they 'bond' with their fetuses while they are still on the inside. When ultrasounds began to receive widespread obstetrical use in the 1980s, scientists studied the efficacy of ultrasound images in encouraging bonding between pregnant women and their babies, and psychologists officially recommended using the technology to help constitute proper maternal attachment.[42] The pregnant woman was thereby taken as sufficiently separate from her insides to need socially ritualized and technologically mediated means for becoming attached to these insides. Pregnant women's widespread acceptance of this goal, and their use of public materials as a means to accomplishing it, indicate that they recognize themselves as required to undergo this bonding on the basis of generic features of the inside of their bodies, rather than on the basis of their interactions with an actual individual child.

The tropes that I have been exploring so far in this chapter are all exemplified elegantly in a recent *Time* magazine cover article entitled "Inside the Womb."[43] The article heralds a "biomedical revolution": the invention of new imaging techniques that give us even more vivid and detailed fetal images than those previously available. This new technology is, as the article puts it, the latest in a series of "remarkable advances" in "imaging technologies that allow us to peer into the developmental process [of pregnancy] at virtually every stage." The article explicitly marks itself as a kind of sequel to Nilsson's *Life* article that appeared thirty-seven years earlier.[44] Somewhat oddly, the text and the images in this article have next to nothing to do with one another. Although the article bills itself as being about these new imaging techniques, it switches after the first two paragraphs to new discoveries concerning the importance of the fetal environment to proper fetal development, and the images and the significance of the technology that produced them receive no further discussion.

The written text recreates and reinforces the standard panic over the vulnerability of the womb to penetrating forces, especially those that have to do with the mother's weakness of the will and her temptations to ingest, and it reinscribes the early modern picture of the uterus as having its own appetites and agency. According to the article, we now have new proof of how important the environment of the womb is to fetal development: We "now" know that "long before a child is born its genes engage the environment of the womb in an elaborate conversation, a two-way dialogue that involves not only the air the mother breaths and the water she drinks but also what drugs she takes, what diseases she contracts and what hardships she suffers." Notice that the conversation here is with the womb, not the mother, who is not one of the agents in this dialectic, even though it is she that is given responsibility for keeping the space of the womb pure. While she is precluded from direct engagement in the dialectic, even her diseases are rhetorically figured here as her active responsibility, by way of the grammar of the active voice—'the diseases *she contracts*.' So the mother, here as hundreds of years ago, is rendered transparent and permeable, but at the same time always potentially blameworthy for her capricious and disorderly temperament and her tendencies to ingest inappropriately: "The list of potential threats to embryonic life is long. It includes not only what the mother eats, drinks or inhales, . . . but also the hormones raging through her body," the article continues. Notice that these 'potential threats' are not marked here as issuing from the environment or economy or health care system that helps determine what a mother 'eats, drinks or inhales,' but from the mother's body itself. One *Time* letter-writer, who identifies herself as a nurse, comments that the article will be helpful in making pregnant mothers take responsibilities for their actions.[45] The images in the article, on the other hand, make no story about the vulnerability of the womb available to the reader's eye. Instead, underscoring the status of the article as a sequel, they recreate Nilsson's tropes with greater vivacity and, under the rhetorical guise of unprecedented realism, help to further entrench and legitimize the official truth about the look of the fetus and its place in the maternal and cultural imagination.

Most of the letters that *Time* magazine published in response to this article focus entirely on the images rather than the text, without showing any cognitive dissonance concerning the mismatch between the two. One pregnant letter-writer calls the photos in the article "our very first photo album." She is more than willing to let a public representation of a generic fetus stand in for her particular child in her family rituals designed to mark and celebrate the identity of that child. Another writes, "I am nine months pregnant . . . this is our first baby (it's a boy) and to see all of what's growing inside of me was a blessing from God."[46] This letter smoothly interprets the public photos as providing visual access to her own insides. The 'this' in her letter seems to refer *both* to the public fetus represented in the article, which she describes as 'what's growing inside of *me*,' *and* to her own version of this fetus, which she marks as male and hence as 'personalized' and not simply generic. These letters reflect the extent to which a canonical, public fetus has become the imaginative measure of each fetus housed in an individual woman's body, as well as the role that the public fetus plays in women's forging individualized bonds with the creature inside of them.

In her 1992 article on public visual representations of fetuses, Janelle Taylor wrote:

> What does the sight of the fetus mean in contemporary American culture? It will be useful to distinguish here between 'personal' images (i.e. ones which a woman might view as representing her own fetus, taken by her own doctor, at her own request and for her own purposes) and 'public' images (representing 'the fetus' and employed outside of the clinical setting, for non-medical purposes).[47]

To whatever extent this distinction was a firm one in 1992, my argument at the moment is that precisely this distinction has interestingly and importantly broken down, as these letters vividly indicate. We simply cannot—and, more importantly, in practice do not—distinguish between private and public representations of fetuses, nor, likewise, between 'my' individual fetus and 'the' generic fetus. The ritualized use of ultrasound and other medical imaging undermines a distinction between images that are taken 'by the woman's own doctor,' 'at her request,' and those that belong in shared, public space. I already pointed out that the production of these images now rarely requires the request, or even the explicit consent, of the pregnant woman. More pointedly, I have been arguing that what Taylor calls representations of 'the fetus' now *are* the representations that individual women use as representations of their own fetuses, and likewise, images that do happen to be of a particular woman's own insides are interpreted and understood through the medium of the public, canonical representations, thereby losing their easy status as 'personal' *as opposed to* public and common. Taylor's correlation of the publicity of an image with its nonmedical use outside of a clinical setting is also hard to sustain now. For instance, medical professionals see public, nonmedical images of generic fetuses as tools for creating personal responsibility and personal commitments to particular fetuses, as we saw in the nurse's response to the *Time* article. Health professionals, advocates, and pregnant women alike use fetal representations as tools for regulating the pregnant body, and we cannot draw a neat line between the medical/clinical use of these representations and their broader cultural use.

THE 'WHAT TO EXPECT PREGNANCY UNIVERSE'

As anyone who has been or lived with a pregnant woman over the last fifteen years knows, *What to Expect When You're Expecting* is the pregnancy guide that has been canonized as *the* official source of pregnancy information—a status that apparently transcends class and race lines. It is the forty-fourth biggest seller on amazon.com,[48] and a third revised edition was recently released. Women routinely pass their copies on to their friends and steal the book from public libraries.[49] The book even shows up in Hollywood movies as a symbol for proper involvement in a pregnancy: In the (insipid) 1995 film *Nine Months*, directed by Chris Columbus, pregnant protagonist Julianne Moore is portrayed as reading *What to Expect When You're Expecting*. Co-star and jilted expectant father Hugh Grant, in the dramatic climax to the movie, tries to convince Moore that he has finally committed himself to being involved in Moore's pregnancy. Moore remains doubtful, until Grant tells her, "I read that book—*What to Expect When You're Expecting*—I read the whole thing from cover to cover." "You did?" Moore asks incredulously, with tears in her eyes . . . and agrees to take him back and accept him as the father of her child. (Significantly, Grant's consumption of public and generic information is here taken as the mark of his commitment to *this particular* pregnancy.) The book is so popular that it has spawned a mini-industry, including a "What to Expect" cookbook; a "What to Expect" pregnancy organizer; two "What to Expect" sequels; a series of "What to Expect" books for kids, with titles such as *What to Expect When You Go to the Potty*; and even send-offs such as *What to Expect When Your Wife's Expanding*. The series increasingly serves as an emblematic target for academic critique as well.[50] One website (now defunct) was dedicated to advertising this set of products collectively, as the "What to Expect Pregnancy Universe." The very fact that there exists a *single* text so canonized strongly contributes to contemporary pregnant women's experiences of their pregnancies as instantiations of a shared and streamlined public event.

The pregnancy organizer is of particular interest.[51] It is nominally a journal or 'planner,' but one that provides a prefabricated structure to the pregnancy narrative and its highlights. It offers slots for the pregnant woman to fill in what she eats, her symptoms, weekly weight, pregnancy milestones, medical information, and so on, as well as suggesting shopping lists and wardrobe essentials. It also asks for descriptions of her psychological and emotional reaction to various events, such as first feeling the baby kick. The detailed structure of the book guides the interpretation and experience of any particular pregnancy, while the blank lines that encourage *you* to fill in *your* individual pregnancy details help the 'organizer' to carry out its individuating function as well. The 'organizer' literally enables you to inscribe *your particular* experiences and narrative, even as it constitutes them in accordance with a public, canonical form. In fact, here the process of 'personalizing' your pregnancy *is* the process of fitting it into such a common form, within which some constrained variations are allowed. Furthermore, the book's marketing presumes that women will take their pregnancies as events in need of such 'organization'; according to the title it is the pregnancy *itself* that gets organized with the help of the book. This harkens back to the calls to 'govern and order' the pregnant body in seventeenth-century guides.

The question-and-answer format of *What to Expect* itself has at least two pertinent rhetorical effects. First, it allows the text to be written in the second person so that the book speaks to *you*, again with the ironic effect of personalizing the pregnancy in and through referring it to generic public representations. Second, it lets the text give determinacy to the half-formed or slightly differently formed questions that pregnant women might have, thereby helping constitute their attitudes and concerns about their pregnancies in line with a common norm. That is, the questions in the text have definite performative force, in the sense that their very articulation not only suggests what questions and concerns are appropriate for pregnant women to have but also creates, shapes, and reshapes readers' prior concerns. Such texts participate in generating and incarnating a canonical, public pregnancy and fetus and function as the media through which women forge an individualized, albeit third person, relationship with their own pregnancies and fetuses.

TRANSPARENCY, ANONYMITY, AND MATERNAL IDENTITY

When Kawana Ashley, a nineteen-year-old low-income pregnant woman, shot herself in the abdomen in Florida in 1997, thereby indirectly killing her six-month-old fetus, who survived the gunshot with minor injuries but died from complications from premature birth, the local newspaper reported that she had "fired a bullet into her womb."[52] Ashley's skin simply vanished, in this representation of the event, leaving no intermediary between her womb and the external world. She was charged with third-degree murder, although the Florida Supreme Court dismissed the charges.[53] I suggest that this representational trope is symptomatic of a larger transformation in our construal of the pregnant body. As a shared pregnancy narrative becomes canonized, and the inside of the pregnant body is transformed into a public arena, the individual outsides of pregnant bodies are rendered permeable and transparent. The anonymous, canonically representable inside of the womb, as it hardens into a familiar form that belongs to and in public space, supplants the character of the pregnant woman herself.

For example, a 1996 medical textbook, *Obstetric and Gynecologic Milestones Illustrated,*[54] begins most of its chapters with a picture of some part of the internal reproductive system, where this picture is the same size as and appears next to a head shot of the research doctor (almost invariably male, with the one exception of Virginia Apgar) who first discovered that feature of the female body and made it public. (On a few occasions, the head shot of the researcher is juxtaposed with a picture of a tool he invented for penetrating the pregnant body.) The visual effect is that these uncased insides of pregnant woman's bodies function as *portraits* of anonymous pregnant insides, to be compared directly with portraits of the men who opened some dimension of these women up to the public eye. Even the layout and framing of the reproductive organs on the page clearly mimics that of the head shot, highlighting the portrait effect (see figure 4.2). Brief biographies of each pictured doctor are included, and the chapters are named after these individual doctors and the body parts they discovered. In the half of the book that covers obstetrics, there is only one photo of the surface of a woman's body.[55] Thus the history of obstetrics is here presented in terms of a litany of medical (and usually male) claimings and displacements into public space of the insides of the pregnant body. The visual contrast here between the anonymity and transparency of the pregnant body, and the named and narrativized (and sometimes literally signed) identity of the individual doctors, is stark, as is the exhibition of the ongoing migration of the inner recesses of the pregnant body outward into the clear and medically owned and managed light of the public world.

Earlier I argued that pregnant women in contemporary North America understand their relationship to their fetuses in and through their third-personal relationship to a public, generic fetus that stands as the interpretive and authenticating measure of their own fetuses. Likewise, pregnant women are encouraged to find their *own* identities in and through these public, generic codifications of their insides. For instance, Georges and Mitchell point out that in the first and second

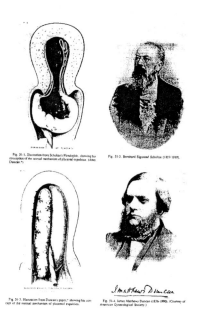

Figure 4.2. Figures 51.1, 51.2, 51.3, 51.4, from Harold Speert, *Obstetric and Gynecologic Milestones Illustrated* (New York: Parthenon, 1996), reprinted courtesy of the publisher.

editions of *What to Expect When You're Expecting,* "Descriptions of each month of pregnancy begin with a drawing of a headless, armless woman, her breast bared and her transparent torso containing only a vagina, rectum, bladder, uterus, and fetus. The caption reads 'What You May Look Like.'[56] The dramatically beheaded and depersonalized depiction of the pregnant body whose insides are a spectacle is notable enough as evidence of the cultural inscription of the transparent pregnant woman and her theatrical uterus (see figure 4.3). But the caption is at least as interesting[57] insofar as it calls upon women to directly identify with this impersonal, dismembered, transparent image of themselves and hence to find their pregnant identities in their spectacularized and fungible wombs (even though they are also asked to have a third-personal, mediated relationship with these wombs and hence, presumably, with themselves). Furthermore, the monthly short description of "what you may look like" that accompanies each drawing, notwithstanding the caption, focuses entirely on the physical features of the *fetus,* such as its size and whether it is coated in downy lanugo or cheesy vernix, so that the 'look' of the pregnant woman is represented as simply identical with the 'look' of a generic fetus at the appropriate stage of gestation. I must admit that as a rhetorically savvy and culturally literate pregnant consumer of *What to Expect* in 2001, I looked at these monthly pictures and captions with no consciousness whatsoever of the absurdity of their message. I examined myself care-

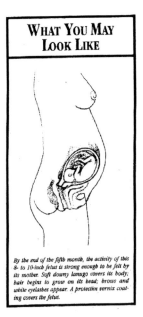

WHAT YOU MAY LOOK LIKE

By the end of the fifth month, the activity of this 8- to 10-inch fetus is strong enough to be felt by its mother. Soft downy lanugo covers its body; hair begins to grow on its head; brows and white eyelashes appear. A protective vernix coating covers the fetus.

Figure 4.3. "What You May Look Like—Fifth Month," from Murkoff et al., *What to Expect When You're Expecting,* 2nd ed. (New York: Workman Publishing, 1996).

fully in the mirror each month, comparing myself—in all my specificity, complete with opaque skin, head, and limbs—as best I could to
the picture, trying to determine whether I had the 'proper look' for my
stage of pregnancy.

Notice that these images of anonymous, schematic, or invisible
pregnant women actually return us to *pre*-Revolutionary representational conventions. Anatomists such as Snip, Hunter, and d'Agoty rein-
stated the fetus within the mother's body in their eighteenth-century
drawings, but these new images resonate instead with those of the seventeenth century that we looked at in chapter 1, when the uterus was
carefully abstracted away from the embodied agent who housed it.
When *the* fetus becomes a shared, public figure, and pregnancy becomes
a canonical narrative, the bodies that house and enact a pregnancy become imaginatively interchangeable. As we did in the seventeenth century, we represent the fetus as self-standing and render the body that
contains it invisible and anonymous. But the motive for this recidivism
is no longer prudery. Rather, the fetus is now in some ways *more* real,
familiar, and public than the surfaces of women's bodies.

CIVIC RESPONSIBILITY, MATERNAL AGENCY, AND THE TECHNIC OF PREGNANCY

We saw in chapters 2 and 3 that there are clear social and medical reasons motivating us, as a culture, to transform pregnancy from a private, unarticulated episode into a public, civic project. I examined at
length how the maternal body and its functioning have enormous
civic importance. As a civic symbol and the site of the civic responsibility for the production of human nature, the maternal body needs to
be a manageable object for policing and regulation. This is impossible
when the insides of the pregnant body are privatized and the process
of pregnancy left to the measure of subjective, idiosyncratic women's
experiences, without any common language and practices for situating
these experiences. Our history of taking the pregnant body as especially permeable, and the womb as especially in need of being kept
pure and protected from the poisoning ingestions of the mother,
heightens our social need to take pregnancy out of the murky shadows
of the private and subjective and into the clear space of objective public discourse, interpretations, and practices. In virtue of their unstable
boundaries, their propensities for hysterical disorder and passion, and
their enormous metaphysical and social responsibility for producing
human nature, pregnant women are inducted into appropriate spaces
and regimes of public body management.

From a civic point of view, the project of pregnancy is the production of well-ordered human nature. When this first became explicit in the eighteenth century, as we saw, the corresponding social rhetoric focused on the importance of producing proper citizens well suited to sustaining a strong and harmonious body politic. Since the eighteenth century we have sustained and intensified our emphasis on what has been labeled 'fetal perfectionism': the idea that mothers have a duty to maximize the potential and future accomplishments of each fetus and child. While the language of the body politic has become somewhat anachronistic, the *civic* interest in fetal perfectionism—a term that resonates perfectly with Rousseau's picture of human nature as 'perfectible'[58]—remains. We demand that mothers regulate the natures of their offspring with precision, and we hold them responsible for any failure to maximize their chances for fetal perfection where there exists public knowledge and personal disciplinary practices whose invocation might increase these chances.[59]

Contemporary mothers are held responsible from the moment of conception for controlling and perfecting their children's IQ, allergies, sense of rhythm, facial structure, freedom from genetic diseases, and much more, through what they eat when they are pregnant and nursing, what music they play during pregnancy and infancy, what feeding implements they use, what dietary supplements they take during early pregnancy, and so on. Black women (who are at risk for passing on sickle cell anemia), Jewish women (who are 'at risk' for passing on the astronomically rare Tay-Sachs disease), and older women (who are at increased risk for having children with Down syndrome and other abnormalities) are among the groups whose pregnancies are especially targeted for heightened surveillance and prenatal testing. More generally, the maternal bodies that are treated as especially dangerous are those that in various ways do not neatly incarnate the canonical pregnancy narrative: those of nonwhite and poor women, unmarried women, women with HIV and other health risks, and women who are above or below the socially acceptable age range for pregnancy, whose purported threat to the well-ordering of the body politic through their wanton and irresponsible reproductive behavior is familiar.

I have been emphasizing the extent to which *mothers* and expectant mothers are construed as the seats of responsibility for the *civic* project of fetal perfectionism. But this language already indicates a philosophically and politically significant gap that needs exploring: if this is a civic project, to or for which mothers are held responsible, then the site of the commitment to and ownership of this project is interestingly ambiguous—should it be located in civic society as a whole, or perhaps in the authorities and authoritative institutions (political, medical, etc.) responsible for sustaining civic society, or should it be located in mothers themselves? On the one hand, I have argued that pregnancy has been importantly co-opted by the public domain, precisely because maternal bodies are not taken to be trustworthy seats of fetal and human production. But on the other hand, I also just pointed out how expectant *mothers* are held responsible for living up to the disciplinary standards of the project of fetal perfectionism, and blamed for their failure to do so, and this seems to plant agency firmly in their hands. We have seen this ambiguity already: during the nineteenth century, we noted in chapter 3, accountability to medical authority and transparency to the medical gaze became part of the practice of responsible *self*-governance for pregnant women.

Whether we construe the project of pregnancy as one of producing well-ordered citizens for the good of the body politic, or as one of perfecting fetal outcome, we treat pregnancy as something that is and ought to be *designed*, and designed in accordance with public, social standards. On the one hand, from a practical point of view, it is still ineliminably the pregnant woman herself who must take on the project of designing her pregnancy, in the sense that she is the one who must discipline her own body and practices and who must purify her womb. Tools such as the *What to Expect* "pregnancy organizer," the fetal movement counters given out by doctors, and online 'calculators' that tell a pregnant woman what she should weigh during each week of gestation are marketed to help her in this project. Even though the uterus has importantly become a public space, and pregnancy has been rendered subject to public regulation, it is still the case that overwhelmingly it is pregnant women who have to be agents *of* this public regulation. After all, in a brute physical sense, we do mostly control our own bodies.

But on the other hand, the *project* of fetal perfectionism is often cast as a public, institutionalized project managed by the scientific community. Harold Speert's 1996 obstetrics and gynecology textbook introduces its section on "circumnatal surveillance" by reporting *of the discipline of research obstetrics* that "as the maternal mortality from obstetrical causes approached the irreducible minimum towards the middle of the twentieth century, the quest for excellence in the newborn intensified."[60] Here this quest is portrayed as one belonging to research obstetricians, even though it is mothers' bodies that are in fact expected to subject *themselves* to regimes of self-discipline and self-monitoring in the name of a personal responsibility for excellence in their children's natures. Appropriately, here, the quest for excellence, which cannot be executed through any direct control of mothers' bodies, is identified with the surveillance of the inside of these bodies—the making public of this inner space. Surveillance furthers the quest for excellence by hysterically displacing the site of fetal production into institutional and scientific space, even if mothers' own practices are marshaled as intermediaries for controlling and improving fetal production within this space.

Now if pregnant women are to function as the agents of fetal production, at the same time as this production is to be conducted under the surveillance and regulation of public authority, then health care institutions, broadly construed, must try to ensure that several conditions are met. First of all, a pregnant woman must be provided with a specific *technic* of pregnancy that will compensate for the inherent untrustworthiness and volatility of her passions, body, and behavior. One pregnancy guide advises, "The management of pregnancy and labor is no different in principle from most other things in life. If something is to be done well, it requires careful thought, meticulous planning, a great deal of practice or training, and the certain knowledge that imperfections can be corrected . . . you will then be able to exert self-discipline and control not only on your emotions but also on your reactions and face delivery with a minimum of fear and distress."[61] We saw in part I that this idea that pregnancy is a process to be *managed* through regimes for bodily self-discipline, especially discipline over the emotions, dates back to at least the early modern era. Furthermore, a pregnant woman must be *inducted* into this technic: she needs not only to understand the public standards of self-discipline and bodily regulation by which her pregnancy is to be designed but also to feel personally responsible for meeting these standards. These standards must make a claim on her behavior; she must take them on as her own and turn herself into the agent of her own supervision and management. Finally, the public pregnancy and fetus must be defined and understood in objective, articulable, and measurable terms: their age and features need to be dated, assessed, and policed using public, standardized tests and technology.

Thus an individual woman's induction into a public understanding of her own pregnancy goes hand in hand with her induction into a set of terms that enables her to design and implement a technic of pregnancy whose progress and success can be established using clear public measures. This induction is a concrete social task, accomplished by way of the kind of care, information, and rhetoric she receives. The canonization of a single public fetal character and a single normative pregnancy narrative importantly supports the establishment of public measures of appropriate pregnancy. As pregnant women are brought to understand their own bodies through the media of these canonical products, this helps foster their willingness and ability to discipline themselves in accordance with such public standards. That is, when we understand our pregnant bodies as *already* belonging to the public domain, and as *already* measured and interpreted through public, common objects and narratives, then we will feel 'naturally' responsible to the public norms and regulations governing this public space and its contents.

As many writers have emphasized, the regimes of self-discipline demanded of pregnant women are imposing indeed.[62] Pregnant women are asked to count fetal kicks daily *and* hourly, record these numbers, and report to medical authorities if the numbers do not meet a precise common norm—a practice that gives pretty much every pregnant woman a terrible scare at least once. Sex and exercise are both to be dispensed in specific positions at specific times. Precision that outstrips any particular scientific evidence is introduced into these regimes in order to encourage quantifiable self-discipline. Pregnant women are advised to gain weight on a very specific schedule: two to four pounds for the first trimester, and one-half to one pound every week after that, until week thirty-six when weight gain should cease[63] (even though recommendations for proper weight gain have swung around wildly over the decades, and no research has affirmed that any particular *schedule* of weight gain has any medical significance). Later, new mothers are asked to do the same with respect to feedings, urinations, and bowel movements and are woken up during the night in the hospital at precise intervals to feed their babies, even if this means waking the baby up too. New mothers are asked to record which breast they began their feedings with, and how long the baby spent at each breast, and they are reprimanded if they fail to successfully implement a regular schedule of feeding according to an alternating pattern of breast-offerings. *What to Expect* has incurred the open hostility of many women with its 'Best Odds Diet' for pregnancy, with its incredibly elaborate rules for eating, huge amounts of food intake required to meet these requirements (paired, of course, with admonitions against gaining too much weight), and its policy of zero tolerance toward 'spontaneous' eating.[64] (Notoriously, *What to Expect* advises, "Every bite counts: Before you close your mouth on a forkful of food, consider, 'Is this the best bite I can give my baby?' If it will benefit your baby, chew away. If it'll only benefit your sweet tooth or appease your appetite, put your fork down.")[65] Pregnant women are also terrorized with extremist rhetoric concerning the risks of alcohol, drugs, and other substances that they may be tempted to ingest. Doctors and pregnancy guides regularly tell women that no amount of alcohol can be acceptably ingested during pregnancy, even though researchers have been unable to find any detrimental effects of alcohol consumption among pregnant women who drink lightly to moderately, as part of a healthy lifestyle rather than as self-medication.[66] Virtually all aspects of a pregnant woman's life are subject to this kind of normative and quantifiable regulation. On the one hand, then, responsibility for keeping their uteruses pure and well-ordered is placed on pregnant women's shoulders, while on the other hand, they are subject to exhaustive, demanding, and precise scripts of self-regulation and provided with elaborate, prefabricated regimens of bodily control that are designed to elicit frightened and diligent compliance from otherwise untrustworthy bodies.

A striking feature of the disciplinary regimes governing pregnant bodies is their appeal to *quantifiable* measures of both pregnant behavior and fetal status. In disciplining herself appropriately, the pregnant woman must turn herself, not only into a publicly regulated object but also into a very specific kind of object of quantifiable public surveillance. This quantificational turn is not surprising. For one thing the technic of pregnancy into which women are inducted needs to be one that can be defined and monitored through objective public measures, and quantificational commensurability is the paradigmatic route to this result. Quantificational measures of behavior, risk, and outcome are unambiguously sharable, allowing pregnant bodies to be compared, assessed, and held to common norms without recourse to murky interpretations. For another thing, quantifiable rules and goals are easier to internalize and follow, and hence they help compensate for the passions and temptations of the volatile pregnant body.[67]

In fact, the imaginative figuring of the fetus and the pregnant body as quantifiable exceeds the details of any particular scientific measures. The canonical gray-tone ultrasound image of the fetus comes complete with tiny white letters and numbers around the edge. These framing numbers make their way into completely nonmedical uses of the ultrasound image, such as a notorious Volvo advertisement from about ten years ago. The ad showed an ultrasound image of a fetus in the classic Nilsson position, surrounded by the canonical obscure tiny numbers and letters, with the caption "Is something inside telling you to buy a Volvo?" This advertisement sparked a minor secondary literature of its own, insofar as it played upon the moral agency of the fetus.[68] Janelle Taylor points out that these numbers visually authenticate the image as a piece of "medical evidence."[69] They also, however, serve to figure the fetus as something that comes part and parcel with a series of measures that chart and interpret its progress and hopefully afford it the stamp of canonical normalcy. For my purposes, it is this inscription of the essential measurability of the fetus that is relevant here, insofar as it gives an aura of precision to the project of disciplining the pregnant body in accordance with a scientific technic of pregnancy.

Several authors, including Barbara Duden, Amy Mullin, Deborah Lupton, Marika Seigel, and Rayna Rapp, have pointed out, more specifically, how medical practices and lay sources of pregnancy advice and information (prominently including *What to Expect*) tend to rhetorically structure their advice around the language of statistical risk, using this language as a tool for managing pregnant women's behavior.[70] In other words, women are encouraged to understand their particular pregnancies in terms of where they fall on various statistical bell curves for various risks and to design their pregnancy regimes around the goal of minimizing their position on these curves. Duden suggests that the *civic* and personal responsibility of the mother is to arrange her life so that she places herself, as much as possible, at minimal risk relative to the public space of pregnant bodies; representations of risk curves thus function as "a summons to normalcy, a warning that she should worry about whether in some characteristic her insides fall outside the normal curve."[71] We know that older women are at an increased statistical risk of having babies with Down syndrome, mothers who drink more than six cups of coffee a day have a 4% higher chance of miscarrying in the first trimester, and so on. Pregnant women are presented with these population statistics and advised to design their behavior in terms of their individual positions with respect to these collective public statistics. I think that the deep point here is that when the technic of pregnancy is designed around these population statistics, it does not merely govern pregnant women's *choices* but also provides them with a self-understanding that individuates them via their statistical position with respect to populations. In this context, individual identities are actually *derivative* upon the identity and character of the populations to which they belong.

Often, the risk information provided is extraordinarily specific; for instance, women who are offered an amniocentesis are given not just specific statistics about their personal chance of having a child with Down syndrome but often also the curve of this risk as maternal age increases, how the possible test outcomes would produce new risk numbers and with what confidence levels, how their risk compares with the population at large and with the population controlled for age, and so forth.[72] Many women take these numbers, considered not just as absolute markers of risk but also as relative risk measurements—which it is their job to minimize insofar as they can be controlled—as emotionally weighty factors governing their choices and confidence within a pregnancy. Amy Mullin, for instance, cites one mother who is very upset that her risk of having a baby with Down syndrome is 1 out of 270, when she would have been quite comfortable with the 1 out of 360 risk that would be normal for her age.[73]

What I find interesting in this kind of reasoning is that it is not risk per se that concerns this woman but her personal risk as it places her on a public, shared bell curve of risk. Furthermore, these risks are so small that the differences between them would be psychologically meaningless were it not for the quantitative comparisons available to her. Thus quantificational and statistical representations of pregnancy *make possible* sets of concerns and ways of delineating choices and goals that simply wouldn't be available to us otherwise.

One would hope that any rational being would largely choose their behavioral regimes based on publicly accessible, testable, objective facts, as opposed to something like their private, untutored intuitions (which I have less than no interest in romanticizing or legitimizing). My point here is more specific. Our representations and deployments of risk and population statistics during pregnancy invite each pregnant woman to understand her idiosyncratic pregnancy *in terms of* her quantifiable position on a common, generic risk curve with public validity and to control her pregnancy by controlling her position relative to these percentiles. Hence quantificational measures can be used as tools for implementing technics of pregnancy in which women mediate their behavior and goals using a canonical pregnant body and pregnancy narrative as the measure of their individual pregnancies.

Pregnant women's self-understandings are constituted in relation to (though of course not mimetic identification with) public narratives and representations of the sorts I have examined. These transformations in self-understanding themselves help to internalize the regulatory and disciplinary practices that bring their bodies in line with public norms. But a crucial part of what I want to bring out here is that this 'internalization' is of a complicated sort. As I suggested at the beginning of this section, women do not simply take on standards of self-discipline that they learn from public forums or medical authorities as their own—nor are they simply coerced and disciplined according to heteronymous standards. Crucially, the disciplinary practices of pregnancy put pregnant women into complex and regulated relations with public authorities. Pregnant women must transform their private experiences and their actions into objective and measurable public information, but they must also hold themselves responsible for the reporting and recording of this information. It is part of what makes us count as a *conscientious* expectant or new mother that we consume public pregnancy information such as guides and websites; carefully document numbers of kicks, urinations, etc.; report these results to the proper authorities; have doctors measure our weight, blood sugar level, and fundus height at prescribed intervals; and so forth. These practices of self-surveillance, quantifiable documentation, and public reporting to proper authorities are part of the regime of *self*-discipline that qualifies our pregnancies as civically responsible: pregnant women engage in practices of self-discipline and bodily management *in and through* authorities and public spaces. First-personal conscientiousness, responsibility, and care are constituted as importantly mediated by third-personal medical authority and surveillance.

This complex intertwining of personal and public discipline comes out exceptionally clearly in a passage culled from a 1932 pregnancy guide. Written when the strength of paternalistic medical authority was less contested, the guide tells us,

> We do know that the way the mother's body works will affect the growth and health of the baby. No matter how much a mother knows, whether she is a doctor, a nurse, a midwife, or a mother who has other children, there is only one way that she can ever be *sure* that her body is doing its best work. That is to be examined by a good doctor as soon as she thinks she might be pregnant and to follow his advice.[74]

Here, pregnant women are instructed that not only proper, responsible pregnant behavior but also proper *knowledge* that the 'body is doing its best work' are essentially mediated through the third-personal space of medical authority and surveillance. The passage makes sure to mention the epistemic importance of this mediation *even in the case where the mother is herself a medical authority*, implying that first-personal authority is *intrinsically* insufficient; indeed, the passage goes out of its way to stress that *no amount* of maternal first-personal knowledge, no matter how legitimately begotten, could be sufficient here.[75]

We would not now be so bold in naming the doctor as the final and absolute court of authority with respect to the knowledge and management of the pregnant body. In contemporary North America we prefer to emphasize private individuals' responsibility for their own behavior and choices, including in the medical arena.[76] But this personal responsibility is taken as conscientious only when it manifests proper internalization of authoritative regimes of self-discipline *and* includes the choice to have one's personal activities mediated and surveyed by medical authorities in public space. So for example, while we now stress women's freedom to choose which prenatal tests they will or won't have, what kind of prenatal medical care they will receive (i.e., whether they will be monitored by a midwife, an obstetrician, or a family doctor), what sorts of pain interventions they will have during childbirth, and so forth, avoiding prenatal medical care altogether or simply not making explicit, medically mediated decisions about these issues is not treated as an acceptable, conscientious choice. Several authors have pointed out the stigma that attaches to mothers (predominantly low-income and socially marginalized mothers) who do not undergo prenatal medical surveillance, even when they have no reason to believe that their pregnancy is medically risky or complicated.[77]

What we see here is a highly complex set of interdependencies and mutually constitutive relationships between personal choice, personal responsibility, public accountability, subjection to authority, self-discipline, and first- and third-personal knowledge. Not only does conscientious pregnancy require a *mixture* of these, but each is *itself* constituted through the others. Taking these complexities seriously means giving up on some entrenched dichotomies within ethics and the metaphysics of the self. We have on our hands a potent object lesson in how little we can assume the adequacy in practice of a simple model of selfhood where responsibility, commitment, and agency can be neatly located and correlated, or where a simple dichotomy between autonomous self-government and paternalistic co-option of agency can be sustained. We can describe women neither as simply the responsible agents of their own pregnancies, nor as merely passive and objectified pawns of paternalistic authority.

It is common for feminist scholars[78] to claim that pregnancy has been treated as a passive state, in which women have been objectified and treated as mere receptacles, and to argue that pregnant women must be reconceived and repositioned as active and agential. For example, Susan Feldman argues that pregnant women have been taken as passive sites of the unfolding of a process that is beyond their control. She suggests that women will be empowered if they understand pregnancy as an active process of 'growing' or 'cultivating' a baby.[79] I hope by now to have shown that this genre of argument is problematic, in at least two senses.

First, while philosophers over the millennia, at least since Socrates, have been fond of such passive receptacle imagery, we have seen that as a matter of empirical fact, pregnant women are expected to take active charge of the outcomes of their pregnancies.[80] Hence they are neither understood nor even allowed to be merely passive spectators with respect to their own pregnancies—they must treat pregnancy as *work* that must be properly designed and executed, and they must exercise *self*-discipline and *self*-management of this active work rather than merely subject themselves to the discipline and management of others. If anything, we have gone overboard in treating babies as needing active, directed 'cultivation' even during gestation. Indeed, we have seen that this vision of pregnancy as an active project, and of the pregnant body as playing an agential role in fetal development, dates back at least to the seventeenth century.

Second, we have seen that the entire dichotomy between passivity and activity, objectification and autonomy, does not function neatly in the case of pregnancy. I have just argued that conscientious pregnant behavior, as currently constituted, requires self-discipline and personal choice and work, essentially mediated through medical authorities and public spaces, and that the pregnant body is importantly positioned as a site of both public, civic investment and personal responsibility. Thus the goal of transforming pregnancy, or our conception of pregnancy, *from* something passive and objectified *to* something active and autonomous already problematically oversimplifies the constitution of pregnant agency, responsibility, and authorship, which cannot be thought of as falling somewhere on a *continuum* from passivity and heteronomy to activity and autonomy in the first place. We cannot confuse the displacement of the fetus into public space, and of pregnancy into civic space, with the passivity or the objectification of the pregnant body. We need to think about pregnancy as situated within a subtler and richer moral and political terrain—and even, I would claim, as requiring a subtler and richer ontology of the self—in order to grasp its ethical shape.

MATERNAL DUTIES AND THE CONSTITUTIVE POWER OF IDEOLOGY

It is tempting to think that all of the advice and information and regimes that pregnant women negotiate is simply the by-product of new medical advances that aid the health of children and the societies that support them. Indeed, it is important never to lose sight of the concrete medical benefits enabled by contemporary technics of pregnancy. Our current surveillance and regimentation of pregnant bodies has enabled advances in fetal, infant, and maternal health and possibilities that were formerly inconceivable. My analysis in this chapter of the publicization and discipline of the pregnant body, taken as the body of the Unruly Mother, should in no way be construed as a plea for a counter-ideology of pregnancy as properly protected from interference and left to take its 'natural' course, or placed in the hands of 'maternal intuition.'[81] Indeed, I have already criticized the ideology of the 'natural' maternal body in earlier chapters, and I will return to this critique in the next chapter.

We need to remember, however, that the regimes that regulate pregnant bodies, and our belief in the special permeability of women's boundaries and their special susceptibility to the dangers of ingestion, transcend the particular medical lore and recommendations that give content, at different times, to these regimes and beliefs. The required regimens controlling the weight gain, feeding practices, nutrition intake, exercise routines, and so forth for the maternal body change almost yearly. Whether or not the current recommendations are closer to being objectively appropriate than were past recommendations, it is important to recognize that almost no other bodies receive the kind of regulation, quantification, and public scrutiny that pregnant bodies do. Despite their real medical benefits, our surveillance and discipline of pregnant bodies has upheld an ethos of these bodies as the privileged, even exclusive sites of civic responsibility, often at the direct and tragic cost of sufficient attention to the many other crucial determinants of maternal and child health that lie outside of the boundaries of the pregnant body, such as domestic violence, environmental damage, and the ravages of poverty.

Yet at the same time, one feature of the ideological practices that constitute and manage the pregnant body that I find most compelling is that they are not the kind of practices that we can simply or morally just think our way out of. We sometimes call something an 'ideology' in order to suggest that if we see through it, and reveal it as a product of cultural pressures and representations rather than as a 'natural given,' then we will be able to escape from its claims over our thought and actions. Whether or not this is ever actually the case with any ideology worth its salt, it is not the case here. The transformation of the uterus into a public theater and of the fetus into its canonical lead actor has come along with the availability of a wealth of information that can help us to improve the capacities and the chances for flourishing of our future children. It seems to me that it is next to impossible not to understand the new availability of such information as constituting some genuine moral duties on our part to obtain it, and to discipline ourselves appropriately in light of it.

It is a moral problem of the first order of difficulty to figure out exactly what the shape and reach of these duties are; it is by no means obvious how to come up with an ethical account that resists demanding unlimited self-sacrifice and discipline from mothers, and at the same time resists turning a blind eye to any moral claims that interrupt a mother's bodily liberty. But despite this difficulty, it seems to me that we simply cannot defend the idea that the information and representations provided to pregnant women are morally neutral or irrelevant. The *accessibility* of such information and representations makes substantive moral claims upon an expectant mother, who must make decisions about how to act and what to find out during pregnancy. How could it be morally unproblematic to act in a way that we know substantially decreases our chances of having a healthy, flourishing baby, and how, even, could it be free of moral complications to choose not to avail ourselves of information that could help us act so as to increase these chances? Once we have made the decision to see a pregnancy through and bring a child into the world, I cannot imagine how enabling the future well-being of that child could fail to constitute a crucial (albeit complicated) moral project for us.

Here I part ways with Barbara Duden, for instance, who is willing to insist that contemporary attempts to discipline the behavior of pregnant women and to publicize their insides are straightforward violations of these women's rights.[82] This attitude seems to me to rely on an unacceptably coarse ontology of selfhood and of rights—one that takes the pregnant woman as an unproblematically bounded and constituted agent with a straightforward set of rights protecting her autonomy, rather than as an agent whose very nature and boundaries are themselves under contest during pregnancy. The pregnant woman is in the midst of transforming from one being into two beings, who are themselves not morally independent of one another but deeply and intimately bound to one another in complex, ethically subtle ways. Our fetuses are not independent agents, but they are not simply more of us either.

The ideology of the surveillance, management, and discipline of the body of the Unruly Mother is not just a body of discursive propaganda but a set of practices that has initiated genuine advances in what we can do to protect and promote the flourishing of our future children, and these advances have moral import. But just because an ideology constitutes *real* moral duties and possibilities does *not* make it any less of an ideology. And such an ideology and its effects can be problematic and worthy of serious critical attention, even once the real moral pressures it constitutes have already been set into motion. We need to be critically aware of how the practices and representations that configure contemporary pregnancy presuppose and buttress a specific ontology and ethics of the pregnant body, articulating its boundaries and its possibilities, and shaping women's first-person understandings and experiences of their own pregnancies.

Perhaps we ought to remind ourselves here that when subjects constitute their identities *in and through* public representations, this does not mean that they simply and mimetically *internalize and recreate* these public representations. We always negotiate and respond to representations of our identity across some critical distance, and pregnant subjectivity and identity are no exceptions. Pregnant women are usually—albeit in varying degrees—somewhat resistant and noncompliant when it comes to socially institutionalized demands upon their behavior and self-conception. But even if we understand ourselves through the (partial) rejection or subversion of public demands and representations, we are thereby importantly marked and constituted by these demands and representations and not merely un-fettered by them. For instance, while women often bond, during and after pregnancy, over how 'silly' or 'manipulative' they found *What to Expect When You're Expecting*, they also recognize it as a shared text that provides them with a set of meanings, norms, and representations serving as a public touchstone for their individual interpretations and experiences of contemporary pregnancy: one that has crucial effects despite—and even through—women's resistance to it and noncompli-ance with its demands.

We cannot understand the ethical or the ontological power of im-ages and other representations of pregnant bodies to co-opt pregnant women's self-understandings unless we recognize the enormous volatility of our self-images and senses of identity during pregnancy. Almost every dimension of a woman's identity needs to be overhauled, transformed, and rebuilt during pregnancy: her social position, her time, her economic habits and status, her body image, her relations to others both passing and intimate, and last but not least, her embodied negotiation of and motion through the material world.[83] Other than dramatic major illnesses and early infancy, there are no other periods of our life during which our bodily shape, capacities, and sensations change so rapidly and dizzyingly. Our normal enjoyment of a lived sta-bility that makes possible other normal negotiations of the world draws upon the fact that we usually look more or less the same each time we look in the mirror and that we can count on our clothes and chairs and cars fitting us more or less the same way, our limbs and or-gans responding predictably, and so on. During pregnancy, we are forced to find ways of not only negotiating but also *re*negotiating our social, economic, personal, and public identity, projects, and relation-ships, at the very same time as our most basic and concrete sense of our bodily self is changing at breakneck speed.

I began this book by pointing out our long history of figuring the pregnant body as especially fluid and unstable. This picture is rife with mythic and ideological dimensions; however, I think it is worth holding onto the concrete sense in which this instability is real and poses a pragmatic challenge to the pregnant woman. There are femi-nist critics who will be distressed by my construing pregnancy as an 'abnormal' state, for many have worked hard to reclaim the normalcy of pregnancy, against the background of a history of treating it as a de-fect or a disease.[84] But I insist that we will not understand what is at stake in representing the pregnant body unless we acknowledge an important dimension of abnormality—of lived *uncanniness*—to con-temporary pregnancy, which after all takes up no more than a couple of years of most women's lives in our culture and is far from static during that time.

In fact, I would argue that the mundane and unavoidable volatility and uncanniness of the pregnant body and self are both crucial to enabling the elaborate social transformations and contestations of the nature and boundaries of pregnant bodies and crucial to understanding the political and ethical significance of these transformations and contestations. During normal conditions, we enjoy much more entrenched and resilient senses of self, which are less plastic in the face of changing public representations and understandings. It make sense that when we are fundamentally struggling to get our bearings, on the other hand, external representations and images that provide us with public touchstones for our identity, with established meanings and uses, would be especially compelling. Likewise, it is during these periods of transition that our sense of self can most easily be co-opted; this is when we are most vulnerable to public constructions that ultimately jeopardize our healthy boundaries and our integrity and autonomy. Hence we need to direct our most careful analytic attention to rhetoric, representations, and practices that configure such vulnerable and plastic selves.[85]

NOTES

1. See chapter 1.

2. John Elkinton, Penguin Books.

3. Roger Stevenson, *The Fetus and Newly Born Infant: Influences of the Prenatal Environment* (St. Louis: Mosby Co., 1973).

4. S. Markens, C. Browner, and N. Press, "Feeding the Fetus: On Interrogating the Notion of Maternal-Fetal Conflict," *Feminist Studies* 23, 1997, 351, my emphasis.

5. Quoted at Markens et al., 358.

6. See especially H. Murkoff, S. Hathaway, and A. Eisenberg, *What to Expect When You're Expecting*, 2nd ed. (New York: Workman Publishing, 1996).

7. This cultural mythos gives context to the self-description of one mother hospitalized for obsessive-cultural disorder specific to pregnancy: "I came to believe that every familiar object was contaminated in some way—food, crockery, cutlery, clothes, sheets, books and so on. The world was swarming with harmful bacteria that I couldn't control or eradicate." (E. Bellamy, "Mother Love Gone Wrong," *The Weekend Australian Review*, March 21, 1998, 16–17).

8. See Katha Pollit, "'Fetal Rights': A New Assault on Feminism," in *'Bad' Mothers: The Politics of Blame in Twentieth Century America*, ed. Ladd-Taylor and Umansky (New York: New York University Press, 1998), 290.

9. Pollit 1998, 287.

10. For documentation of this, see for instance Jennifer Terry, "The Body Invaded: Medical Surveillance of Women as Reproducers," *Socialist Review* 19, 1989.

11. Barbara Duden, *Disembodying Women: Perspectives on Pregnancy and the Unborn*, trans. L. Hoinacki (Cambridge: Harvard University Press, 1993), 81.

12. See for instance Linda Blum, *At the Breast* (Boston: Beacon Press, 1999), 59–60; Emily Martin, *The Woman in the Body: A Cultural Analysis of Reproduction* (Boston: Beacon Press, 1987); and Naomi Wolf, *Misconceptions: Truth, Lies and the Unexpected on the Journey to Motherhood* (New York: Doubleday Books, 2001).

13. Lisa Mitchell, *Baby's First Picture* (Toronto: University of Toronto Press, 2001), 26.

14. National Public Radio, Washington, DC, October 2002.

15. See for instance Duden 1993; Rosalind Pollack Petchesky, "Fetal Images," *Feminist Studies* 13, 1987; Janelle Taylor, "The Public Fetus and the Family Car: From Abortion Politics to a Volvo Advertisement," *Public Culture* 4, 1992; and Deborah Lupton, "Risk and the Ontology of Pregnant Embodiment, in Lupton, ed., *Risk and Sociocultural Theory* (New York: Cambridge University Press, 1999).

16. See, among many other examples, Petchesky 1987; Taylor 1992; Duden 1993; Rayna Rapp, *Testing Women, Testing the Fetus* (New York: Routledge, 1999); Barbara Katz Rothman, *The Tentative Pregnancy: Prenatal Diagnosis and the Future of Motherhood* (New York: Penguin, 1987); and Eric Parens and Adrianne Asch, eds., *Prenatal Testing and Disability Rights* (Washington: Georgetown University Press).

17. L. Michaels and M. Morgan, eds., *Fetal Subjects, Feminist Positions* (Philadelphia: University of Pennsylvania Press, 1999) is a good example of a prominent anthology on this topic that is entirely structured around the politics of exceptional pregnancies.

18. Duden 1993, 7.

19. Harrison et al., "Management of the Fetus with a Correctable Congenital Defect," *Journal of the American Medical Association* 246, 1981, 774. Quoted at Petchesky 1987, 276.

20. My thanks to Sarah Hardy for pointing out the absurdity of the size of the fetus, which would be as large as a schoolchild if its proportions were accurate.

21. Duden 1993, 14.

22. Indeed, women are (rightly) told that their own tactile assessments of quickening are not trustworthy and that they might at first mistake gas and other minor gastronomic disturbances for fetal movement, or vice versa; ultrasounds are now the official measure of the life and age of the fetus.

23. I will have much more to say later on what I mean precisely by calling this identity 'quantifiable.'

24. Lisa M. Mitchell and Eugenia Georges, "Cross-Cultural Cyborgs: Greek and Canadian Women's Discourses on Fetal Ultrasound," *Feminist Studies* 23:2, 1997.

25. Mitchell and Georges 1997, 147.

26. Weir, "Pregnancy Ultrasound in Maternal Discourse," in *Vital Signs: Feminist Reconfigurations of the Bio/Logical Body*, ed. M. Shildrick (Edinburgh: University of Edinburgh Press, 1998), 84, 92.

27. Karen Stohr reminded me that, in fact, ultrasound measurements of the fetus are now the final court of appeal for the due date of a baby, and that as far as official medical records are concerned, this due date will trump even the mother's report that the date is inconsistent with her sexual activity. During my first pregnancy, an ultrasound technician informed me that I was six weeks pregnant a full eight weeks after my first positive pregnancy test, and the gestational age he generated continued to provide the basis for my 'official' due date.

28. Mitchell and Georges 1997, 377.

29. Mitchell 2001, 93.

30. Mitchell 2001, 381.

31. Mitchell 2001, 142.

32. See Mitchell 2001, chapter 1.

33. Thanks to Annie Lyerly for passing on this advertisement.

34. Indeed, Mitchell (2001) shows that many women are excited about their ultra-sounds and want them very badly, even while they are unable to describe any diagnostic purposes of the tests.

35. Mitchell 2001; Rapp 1999.

36. As one friend and colleague who recently experienced a first trimester fetal death put it to me, "I hopped up on the table [for my ultrasound] all ready and excited to see my baby, and then I suddenly had to change my understanding of the situation I was in and the meaning of the event right on the spot." See also Lisa Mitchell, "Women's Experiences of Unexpected Ultrasound Findings," *Journal of Midwifery and Women's Health* 49, 2004, 228–34.

37. Mitchell 2001, chapter 2.

38. For example, at kidshealth.org/parent/system/medical/prenatal_tests.html, the maternal blood screening or 'triple-marker' test, which can reveal a heightened prospect of Down syndrome or neural tube defects and does require signed consent, is listed as one of the 'routine' tests and introduced simply with the comment that "most mothers will have" this test.

39. Weir 1998, 82.

40. www.babycenter.com, December 31, 2002.

41. Eugenia Georges and Lisa M. Mitchell, "Baby Talk: The Rhetorical Production of Maternal and Fetal Selves," in *Body Talk: Rhetoric, Technology, Reproduction*, ed. Lay, Gurak, Gravon, and Myntti (Madison: University of Wisconsin Press, 2000).

42. A classic source is J. C. Fletcher and M. I. Evans, "Maternal Bonding in Early Fetal Ultrasound Examinations," *New England Journal of Medicine* 308(7), 1983, 382–83. For a recent renewed interest in this issue in the context of the enhanced bonding opportunities offered by 3-D ultrasound images, see I. E. Timor-Tritsch and L. D. Platt, "Three-dimensional Ultrasound Experience in Obstetrics," *Current Opinion in Obstetrics and Gynecology*, 14(6), 2002, 569–75.

43. November 11, 2002.

44. The images come from the work of Alexander Tsiaras, and the article coincided with the publication of his book, *From Conception to Birth: A Life Unfolds* (New York: Doubleday, 2002). This work is being routinely discussed as a sequel to Nilsson's, and Tsiaras, who describes his images as a combination of art and science, has to a large extent chosen to stick to Nilsson's aesthetic conventions of fetal representation.

45. *Time* Magazine, December 1, 2002.

46. Both letters are from the December 1, 2002, issue of *Time*.

47. Taylor 1992, 69.

48. As of September 2004.

49. Approximately 75% of the dozens of copies of the book in the public library system of Prince George's County, MD (one of the two main suburban DC counties in Maryland) are listed as "long overdue."

50. See for instance Mitchell and Georges 2000; Lupton 1999; and Helen Michie, "Confinements: The Domestic in the Discourses of Upper-Middle Class Pregnancy," in S. H. Aiken et al., eds., *Making Worlds: Gender, Metaphor, Materiality* (Tucson, AZ: University of Arizona Press, 1998), 258–73, as well as this book of course.

51. Eisenberg, Murkoff, and Hathaway, *What to Expect When You're Expecting Pregnancy Organizer* (New York: Workman Publishing, 1995).

52. This language was repeated several times. See for example www.linda .net/kawana.html.

53. A similar point about the reporting of the Kawana Ashley case is made in Susan Squier's "Fetal Subjects and Maternal Objects: Reproductive Technology and the New Fetal/Maternal Relation," *Journal of Medicine and Philosophy*, 21:5, 1996, 515–535.

54. Harold Speert, *Obstetric and Gynecologic Milestones Illustrated* (New York: Parthenon Publishing Group, 1996).

55. In fact, this is not a picture of a pregnant woman but a photo of the naked body of a patient recovering from a cesarean section that utilized breakthrough techniques.

56. Georges and Mitchell 2000, 189.

57. Interestingly, the just-released third edition of *What to Expect* has replaced these captions with ones that read "A Look Inside." I don't know what the motivation was for the change. The authors have declined to comment.

58. See chapters 2 and 3.

59. See Lupton 1999 for an extended discussion of this point.

60. Speert 1996, 265. I here relegate to this footnote the disturbing fact that once maternal *mortality* had been more or less conquered, Speert suggests, attention turned exclusively to *fetal* excellence, as opposed, for example, to improving maternal health. Apparently, failure to die is still the digital measure of the medical success of the pregnancy for the mother.

61. Gordon L. Bourne, *Pregnancy* (New York: Harper and Row, 1975), 18. Many thanks to Marika Seigel for bringing the quotation to my attention.

62. See in particular Lupton 1999 and Michie 1998.

63. See for example *What to Expect When You're Expecting* (Murkoff et al. 1996).

64. Despite its huge sales, *What to Expect* receives an average 'user review' of only three stars out of five on amazon.com. The majority of the user reviews mention their anger at the 'Best Odds Diet' (which suggests a whole-grain muffin for those rare occasions where you can't help but 'cheat' on your diet) as one of their main reasons for withholding a high rating from the book.

65. Murkoff et al. 1996, 81.

66. See Elizabeth Armstrong, *Conceiving Risk, Bearing Responsibility: Fetal Alcohol Syndrome and the Diagnosis of Moral Disorder* (Baltimore: Johns Hopkins University Press, 2004) for an excellent and exhaustive discussion of the inflated hysteria surrounding alcohol consumption during pregnancy. The extremist recommendations that pregnant women face concerning their ingestions of all sorts, but especially alcohol, and the way that these 'recommendations' are conveyed, enforced, and internalized, is an important and complicated topic in its own right that deserves separate discussion. This exploration would take me too far off track here, even though it is closely relevant to the thesis and discussion of this chapter.

67. The quantificational pressures and regimentation facing pregnant bodies have been discussed in several places, that is, in Lupton 1999; Duden 1993; Taylor 1992; Rapp 1998; and Amy Mullin, *Reconceiving Pregnancy and Childcare* (New York: Cambridge University Press, 2005), although my explanation of the purposes of this quantification is somewhat different from that given elsewhere.

68. Taylor 1992; Petchesky 1987; Duden 1993.

69. Taylor 1992, 76.

70. See Rapp 1998; Mullin 2005; Lupton 1999; Duden 1993; and Marika Seigel, "Visualizing and Individualizing Risk During Pregnancy" (presented at the Society for Literature and Science meeting, Durham, NC, October 2004).

71. Duden 1993, 29.

72. See Rapp 1999, for example.

73. Mullin 2005.

74. The Maternity Center Association of New York 1932, 15. I cited this passage in chapter 3 as well.

75. While the passage is surprisingly progressive in mentioning the possibility that expectant mothers may be doctors, the doctor who can give the pregnancy the proper stamp of responsible behavior and certain knowledge is identified with the male pronoun.

76. The post-1960s explosion of medical concern with informed consent is an example of this emphasis. In "Who Will Live? Parents Facing Ethical Dilemmas in Neonatal Intensive Care Units in France and the United States" (presentation, American Society for Bioethics and the Humanities annual meeting, Montreal, October 2003), Kristina Orfali argues for the specificity of this rhetorical orientation to North America.

77. See for example Lupton 1999 and Pollit 1998.

78. See for example Mullin 2005; Lupton 1999; and in particular Susan Feldman, "From Occupied Bodies to Pregnant Persons," in *Autonomy and Community: Readings in Contemporary Kantian Social Philosophy*, ed. J. Kneller and S. Axinn (Albany: SUNY Press, 1998).

79. Feldman 1998.

80. Philosophers are so used to thinking about pregnancy in terms of the passive metaphors that they have inherited from other philosophers, that even when they try to reclaim pregnancy as active they often struggle to find recherché examples of pregnant activity that do not do much violence to these metaphors, instead of pointing out the utterly mundane activities that make up the project of pregnancy, such as showing up for prenatal visits, exercising, taking tests, counting kicks, buying baby supplies, preparing food, reading, and so forth. For instance, Mullin 2005, drawing on similar points by Hilde Lindemann Nelson, tries to underscore the active dimension of pregnancy by pointing out that pregnant women choose to remain pregnant, are emotionally involved in their pregnancies, 'imagine' and 'welcome' their babies, and so forth. This list of 'activities' is quite remarkable in its focus on emotional and mental rather than gross physical activities. As a philosopher, I accept that such mental actions count as genuine actions, but only in a relatively subtle sense. It is interesting that Mullin and Nelson feel that they need to be so subtle in coming up with examples of the activities of pregnancy.

81. For an example of such a move, see Wolf 2001.

82. See Duden 1993, throughout.

83. The classic article on the phenomenology of pregnant embodiment is Iris Young's "Pregnant Embodiment: Subjectivity and Alienation," *Journal of Medicine and Philosophy* 9, 1984, 45–62. While her analysis is a very useful touchstone, she seems to underplay the totalizing and concretely challenging nature of the experience of pregnancy.

84. See for example Feldman 1998.

85. I will return to the political significance of this vulnerability and volatility in my concluding chapter.

5

Separation Anxiety

In chapters 2 and 3, I argued that the culture of the Enlightenment bestowed upon the nursing maternal body the power and the responsibility to create and sustain an appropriate, natural social order. Recent history has sustained and reinforced the Rousseauian vision of the civic capacities and responsibilities of the maternal breast. In 1958, D. W. Winnicott, influential founder of psychoanalytic "object relations" theory and proponent of "attachment parenting" reminded mothers that through the "natural process" of breastfeeding "you are grounding the health of a person who will be a member of our society."[1] In 1971, Ashley Montagu likewise appealed to both the natural significance and the founding social role of the nursing maternal body: "We see how beautifully designed the suckling of the baby at the mother's breast is . . . to serve the most immediate needs of both. . . . What is established in the breastfeeding relationship constitutes the foundation for the development of all human social relationships."[2] Shortly before Michael Moore's notorious exposé of General Motors' corrupt labor practices in Flint, Michigan, the company nicknamed itself "General Motors, the Breast that Feeds Flint."[3] A 1995 article entitled "Nursing the World Back to Health" reinstates the social responsibilities and nostalgic powers of the maternal breast.[4] In 1997, the American Academy of Pediatrics issued a policy statement that proclaimed the "benefits of breastfeeding to the infant, the mother and the nation."[5] In 2004, the United States Department of Health and Human Services, having officially decided that "increasing the proportion of mothers who breastfeed their babies is one of . . . our nation's objectives for improving public health," hired the Ad Council (a private company that brought us Smokey Bear, McGruff the Crime Dog, and the slogan "Friends Don't Let Friends Drive Drunk"} to design a new national campaign to encourage breastfeeding. In a June 4, 2004, press release, Health and Human Services announced that the new campaign tag line would be "Babies were born to be breastfed"—thereby reinforcing the idea that mothers who do not breastfeed thwart the normative, proper natural order. According to the press release, public service announcements structured around this slogan "will be distributed to 28,000 media outlets nationwide and will run and air in advertising time and space that is donated by the media."[6]

In the preceding chapter, we saw how various practices work to spatially displace the fetus from the pregnant body, and how this helps to enable the surveillance and regulation of the maternal environment. Thus, in the language of part I of this book, we saw how expectant mothers' bodies are practically treated as potentially unruly. Given this current institutional entrenchment of the Unruly Mother, one might think that the Fetish Mother who held such iconographic and ideological sway at the end of the eighteenth century is an anachronism. But in fact the body of the Fetish Mother—the maternal body construed as an inarticulate, extended union of mother and infant, joined at the breast and through the milk—still operates as a powerful ideological figure in contemporary North American culture. Just as fears of the corrupting power of the unruly maternal body, with its undisciplined and permeable boundaries and its potentially impure womb, have lasted and taken on new forms in contemporary culture, likewise the restorative and ordering powers of the fetishized lactating maternal body, and her status as a symbol of normative nature, have been re-entrenched and reinvigorated in contemporary practices and rhetoric surrounding early motherhood. The lactating maternal body is still granted the power and the responsibility to *create proper nature*, including a natural social order, although only when it meets mythic standards of 'natural' purity and unity with the infant.

The relationship between the ideological status of the Fetish Mother and the concrete practices concerning actual breastfeeding bodies is complicated, as we will see—now as in the nineteenth century, actual bodies are not simply identified with the Fetish Mother but rather governed by its normative force in complex, mediated ways. While the body of the Fetish Mother founds the moral, psychological, and physical health of individual and social bodies '*naturally*,' real maternal bodies regularly fall short and require various kinds of regulation and intervention; they can by no means be counted upon to fulfill this natural function. I will examine how the proximate, nursing body of the Fetish Mother functions as an ideal that sets up a logic governing the practices, attitudes, expectations, and representations surrounding breastfeeding and the messy bodies that imperfectly realize this ideal. In chapter 3, I tried to show how separations between the bodies of mothers and their infants were represented as hysterical and monstrous schisms that disrupt and deform nature. In this chapter, I examine how this logic of natural proximity and monstrous separation has become a governing trope in our social and scientific representations of early mothering and infant feeding. I examine the contemporary manifestations of the ideological figure of the Fetish Mother and her extended body, which is joined to that of her infant through the bond of milk, through the practices surrounding breastfeeding—I look at how women receive information about breastfeeding, what kind of help or hindrances they face in establishing and continuing breastfeeding, how breastfeeding figures as an object of scientific study and concern, how women are expected and encouraged to feel about breastfeeding, and how they in fact respond to all of these social interventions.

There is no question but that breast milk is the healthiest food for infants under most circumstances. We have solid scientific evidence that infants who receive breast milk as their primary food show lower rates of allergies and asthma, are at lower risk for sudden infant death syndrome and diabetes, and tend to have fewer ear infections, to name just a few benefits.[7] I take it as a guiding principle, no longer in need of support, that getting breast milk to infants when possible needs to be an important public health goal. All the same, in the next couple of chapters I will be looking at how the practices and discourse surrounding breastfeeding can subject women to assaults on their integrity, autonomy, and personal boundaries. The ideological figure of the Fetish Mother and its implementation are, I argue, often oppressive and problematic. One of my major goals, in writing these chapters, was to find a means for critiquing breastfeeding ideology that protects the integrity and boundaries of mothers without explicitly or implicitly casting their interests in opposition to those of their children. It is fairly easy to criticize the pro-breastfeeding movement that has hegemony in contemporary medical and public health institutions from the perspective of straightforward rights-based liberal feminism, claiming that this movement works to reduce women's freedom and re-entrench traditional gender and caretaking roles. Such a critique goes no distance toward questioning and reconfiguring the breastfeeding relationship and its social support and discursive representation themselves, with an eye to making breastfeeding a healthier, more sustainable, less oppressive practice. I do not wish to begin with the conflicting rights or interests of mothers and children, or even with this repertoire of ethical tools and oppositions. Instead, I want to ask how to best understand and transform the social practices surrounding infant feeding, governed by the goal of facilitating the joint flourishing of mothers and infants.

PRINCIPLES OF PROXIMITY

In the 1997 revised edition of La Leche League International's manifesto *The Womanly Art of Breastfeeding*, co-founder Mary Ann Cahill tells new and expectant mothers:

> From living in the womb with the umbilical cord supplying all his needs, [the newborn] has progressed to a position outside of, but near, the mother's body. He is meant to be within close proximity of her warm breast and the sound of her voice. It is nature's careful way of providing a transition from the infant's old world to his new one. . . . The all-important mother-child bond replaces the umbilical cord.[8]

Here the relationship between mother and child is figured spatially, in terms of material proximity and nearness, and as a continuation of the material bond of the umbilical cord. This proximity is figured as both natural and appropriate. This relationship of material, spatial proximity between the infant and the maternal body continues to be positioned as the source and symbol of more abstract, appropriate moral and social relations. Furthermore, the material bond of *milk* in particular, and the proximity of the infant's mouth to the mother's breast, functions as the privileged locus of this all-important proximity. Through the natural (and yet easily corruptible) practice of breastfeeding, the maternal body is taken as capable of and responsible for 'restoring' a normative natural order and a unified body politic, while the bond of milk functions mythically as a material arrangement capable of somehow embodying or carrying a moral arrangement.[9]

According to the classic logic of the fetish, as we saw in chapter 3, a fetish is an object that is granted indefeasible, ahistorical intrinsic value. The fetishization of commodities, in Marxist economic theory, covers over the labor that produces those commodities and the social context that helps fix their value, treating them instead as intrinsically desirable and valuable. Likewise, the fetishization of the extended nursing body covers over the labor of mothering and the purposes, material mechanisms, and social history that make nursing valuable. In rhetoric that fetishizes mother-infant proximity, there is a suggestion that mothering, in all its complexity, can be effectively reduced to nearness, and that the value of mothering is somehow contained in this contiguity of bodies. As long as the mother keeps the child at the breast, this mute, inarticulate positioning will 'naturally' constitute the proper 'bond' that is the mark of good mothering and the guarantor of well-ordered nature. In one movement, material proximity is elevated into a moral principle and symbol, while the ethical structure of mothering is demoted to a mute material arrangement. The reduction of mothering to proximity, and of proximity to breast-feeding, belittles the accomplishments and complexity of mothering by reducing it to a static and inarticulate spatial bond.[10]

In her sympathetic and exhaustive history of La Leche League, Julie DeJager Ward writes, "it is perhaps La Leche League's most deeply held tenet that the physical, emotional and psychological health of the baby depend on an early period of *mother-infant proximity,*"[11] and she frequently describes the "principle of mother-baby proximity" as a structuring force governing League policy and attitudes.[12] This principle takes a spatial arrangement as the essence of good, proper, 'natural' mothering, and, as employed in the context of the League, it also substitutes one particular type of proximity—namely breast-to-mouth contact—for proximity in all of its many forms. We will see examples of this double reduction, of mothering to proximity and of proximity to nursing, throughout this chapter, but its implementation in the case of La Leche League is especially explicit. The League's self-described philosophy is "good mothering through breastfeeding," and their manifesto announces, "Breastfeeding is the most natural and effective way of understanding and satisfying the needs of the baby . . . the do-it-yourself kit for learning good mothering."[13] Indeed, in a revealing reversal of common sense, one League newsletter article claims that maternal and infant "attachment behavior *exists for the purpose of insuring proximity.*"[14] Here mothering is not only reduced to proximity, but proximity has become an end in itself, toward which the lived bond between mother and child is a mere means. Similarly, the authors of the 1990 textbook *Counseling the Nursing Mother: A Reference Handbook for Health Care Providers and Lay Counselors* assure the reader that "breastfeeding . . . is *the* physical embodiment of *the* mother-baby relationship after birth."[15] It is not clear what it means to give physical embodiment—especially a *unique* embodiment—to a social relationship, but the reductive and figurative logic here is clear enough.

Over the course of the last century, proximity has been systematically elevated into a privileged principle and symbol of mothering by several parenting movements both marginal and mainstream. In the middle of the twentieth century, object relations theory revised classical Freudian theory by extending our formative psychological development backward into very early infancy. According to object relations

theorists such as D. W. Winnicott and Melanie Klein,[16] primary oneness between mother and infant, crystallized in their spatial proximity through nursing, is the originary human state, and our development into an individual occurs first and foremost in and through our
struggle to separate from our mother's breast. In classic object relations theory, the nursing body is the paradigmatic maternal body and
the fused 'mother-child dyad' is the originary site of human development, while the spatial figure of the proximate breast and its eventual
rejection governs the logic and iconography of the theory. For Klein,
the infant traverses through a set of 'positions' on its way to ego-inde-
pendence, where these positions are construed as relations to the
breast, and for Winnicott, development into an individual involves the
actualization of the 'potential space' between the body of the mother
and the infant.[17]

Where object relations theorists emphasized the process of *separation* from the breast, some psychological literature with a superficially
opposite thrust similarly assigns a privileged role to the spatially configured body of the Fetish Mother. Ashley Montagu made physical contact between mother and infant into the basic principle of normative
mothering, demanding that mothering be recognized as a "direct continuation of the interuterine state."[18] Just earlier, in the 1960s, William
and Martha Sears became enormously popular parenting gurus through
their theory of 'attachment parenting,' whose central thesis was that
"health, physical, spiritual, emotional and moral child development"
could be facilitated "by placing a premium on extended mother-child
physical contact."[19] A slightly different version of the fetishization of
mother-child proximity shows up in the discourse that claims a special,
crucial period of 'bonding' occurs in the first moments of birth. Linda
Blum writes, "In the late 1970's, John Bowlby's work would fuel a . . .
'bonding craze,' which made the first skin-to-skin, breast-to-mouth
contact so critical" to the child's psychological health, and to the
mother's mothering skills, "that mothers feared disastrous consequences if they missed it or were not instantly enthralled."[20] Here
again, we see an elision between proximity and bonding, both taken as
the source and summary of good mothering in all its complexity.[21]

I want to highlight how little the rhetoric here has changed from
Rousseauian rhetoric that used the figure of the extended, continuous
nursing body as the mark of the natural and well-ordered and as the
wellspring of civic virtue. This mythic link between 'naturalness' and
proximity is widespread and receives surprisingly little critical interrogation.[22] Popular and academic literature alike, in a Rousseauian
voice, blames the 'non-natural' elements of contemporary human life,
which include urbanization and working mothers, or more vaguely,

'Western' or 'technocratic' society, for reducing breastfeeding rates by undercutting mothers' 'natural' inclination to breastfeed by way of reducing proximity.[23] Much of the rhetoric in these works is aimed at setting the mother and her 'natural' inclination toward proximity against the forces that would tear her and her infant apart.

Indeed, proponents of so-called 'natural mothering' more or less identify the naturalness of their mothering practices with their maintenance of proximity. Chris Bobel's recent scholarly study of the 'natural mothering' movement makes this connection explicit. She writes, "The natural mother rejects almost everything that facilitates mother-child separation," and "the natural mother recognizes no artificial, socially prescribed division between mother and child. Rather, they operate as one bonded unit."[24] Interestingly, Bobel is appropriately suspicious of the rhetoric of the natural in the 'natural mothering' movement, but she never questions the propriety of the link between nature and proximity, taking their relevance to one another as self-evident. Indeed, the fetishization of proximity is sufficiently pervasive that it takes a bit of imaginative work to isolate this link and make it explicit so that we can notice that it seems empirically and semantically arbitrary

In the ideology of the extended Fetish Mother, it is not just proximity in general, but specifically *maternal* proximity that is accorded a unique, almost sacred role in well-ordering nature. Each of the parenting movements I have discussed stresses over and over again that the replacement or substitution of the *mother's* physical body, even briefly, is the key corruption against which we need to guard. In a section entitled "making a choice," which argues against mothers returning to work even in the face of fairly serious economic need, the La Leche League guide tells readers, "*No one can replace you* as mother. From all evidence, . . . it can be said that the mother is the one most perfectly suited to be a nurturer in the early years."[25] After citing the quotation from Winnicott that I used on page 145, the guide comments: "The only true basis for the relationship of a child to mother and father, to other children, and eventually to society is the first successful relationship between mother and baby."[26] What we see here is not only the emphasis on spatial proximity as the key to proper mothering but also a focus on the *unique* suitability of the mother's body for proximate mothering, along with the move outward from the proximate relationship to the founding of the proper social order, all pinned on the idea that *only* the mother's body can play this role.

Two potential material media of mother-infant proximity, namely the umbilical cord and the milk of the maternal breast, are each frequently taken to represent or even somehow embody the maternal-infant relationship itself. We saw earlier that according to La Leche

League, "The all-important mother-child bond replaces the umbilical cord." In 1945, Helene Deutsch's influential work *The Psychology of Women* contained the claim that "In nursing, the psychic umbilical cord connects the mother's breast and the child's mouth."[27] In Jellife and Jellife's signal pro-breastfeeding medical anthropology text written in 1978, the infant is referred to as an "extero-gestate foetus."[28] A recent scholarly article states as self-evident fact that "at birth, the infant extends his interuterine dependence to the external comfort of the mother's breasts."[29] This set of metaphors, analogies, and figures inscribes both the *uniqueness* of a particular maternal body for mothering, as well as the brute materiality of the maternal bond. At the same time, it also uses metaphors and figures of *biological* connection (pregnancy, lactation, umbilical cords) to identify, imagine, and demarcate the maternal body. This use of biology surely does grave injustice to the maternal bodies and labor of nonbiological mothers— adoptive mothers, stepmothers, etc.—and this is a crucial topic worthy of its own analysis, which I will just point toward here.

Amy Mullin points out that our frequent practice of treating pregnancy as analogous to (or a preview of) motherhood sets up a framework within which exclusive caregiving relationships are taken for granted: "The tight association between childbearing and childrearing . . . tends to suggest that one person should be a child's primary caregiver, since only one person can have been pregnant with that child."[30] This naturalization of the notion of a primary caregiver helps to grant, prima facie, unthematized plausibility to the notion that the maternal body has unique capacities and bears unique responsibilities. Furthermore, figuring these responsibilities as responsibilities for proximity, on the model of the continuation of pregnancy, turns caregiving into a dyadic and simple relationship without enough articulation or space for social critique or community participation. But we need to remember that the isolation of infants with a single caregiver or even a single feeder who is also their mother is a relatively modern social invention. In chapter 2, we saw that the practice of sending children to wet nurses was completely standard in most European cultures until the eighteenth or nineteenth centuries. This practice separated the larger social role of mothering from the specific task of being a proximate body for an infant. Many cultures share the work of physically caring for infants among a community of women, breaking the bond of uniqueness.[31]

As we saw, it was only in the wake of Rousseau and the Revolution that institutional and social pressures turned against the routine use of wet nurses and artificial feeders.[32] The romantic image of a primitive or peasant society where mothers automatically breastfeed their children for years, in an exclusive, spatially proximate relationship, is a creation of Rousseauian eighteenth-century sentimentalism and a product of the rise of the nuclear family and a specific kind of domestic space. Pam Carter points out that our culture, including feminist culture, has been reluctant to question "the story of the stolen art of breastfeeding."[33] Breastfeeding is regularly called a 'lost' art—the whole phrase "the lost art of breastfeeding" yields enough Google hits to easily establish its status as a slogan. But it is important to remember that the frequent appeals, from Rousseau through to contemporary parenting and breastfeeding literature, to a utopic past, in which a unique and sustained breastfeeding relationship between mother and infant was automatic and unproblematic, invoke a mythical, nostalgic era with no particular literal referent.[34]

MONSTROUS SEPARATIONS

When proximity becomes the touchstone for the proper figuring and functioning of the maternal body, likewise the material separation of mother and infant becomes a breach in the maternal body—one that threatens to undermine the very order of nature. The privileging of proximity correspondingly raises the specter of disaster should this spatial contiguity be interrupted—by a bottle, a pump, a working mother who sends her child to daycare, an HIV infection that contraindicates breastfeeding, an NICU life-support system, a nipple guard, or any number of other interruptions that corrupt the body of the extended Fetish Mother.[35] Indeed, such instruments of interruption are accorded special demonic powers in the rhetoric surrounding early motherhood. And just as the proximate bond between mother and infant is figured biologically, so are the threats and dangers of even passing separation. Psychologist Humberto Nagera writes, "the term 'separation anxiety' . . . refers to the *biological unity* that exists between the mother and the infant, a unity that, if disturbed, leads . . . to very unwelcome results in the development of the child. It must be clear in this case we are referring not only to permanent separations but to transitory ones, separations that may last just a few hours."[36]

Modern manuals such as *What to Expect When You're Expecting* and *So That's What They're For: Breastfeeding Basics*,[37] along with La Leche League's *The Womanly Art of Breastfeeding*, tell mothers that even *one single suck* on an artificial nipple—a bottle or a pacifier—may well destroy their possibilities for breastfeeding forever by inducing 'nipple confusion' and making the infant unwilling to take a 'real' nipple ever again. Even nipple shields are sometimes treated as *morally* dubious, and this is so even when they make possible an otherwise unsuccessful breastfeeding relationship. For instance, Kathryn McPherson, the editor of *The Reality of Breastfeeding: Reflections by Contemporary Women*, writes "I wanted to breastfeed and I was willing to use that *piece of plastic* if I had to, but I *knew it wasn't right.* Why did I have to use this *apparatus?*"[38] This comment nicely illustrates the totemic status of the nipple shield as an emblem of separation and artificiality. The ethical significance that has been cathected onto a simple mechanical aid here is clear, as is the prethematized idea that such a device intervenes upon a process that is supposed to be 'natural' in a normative sense.

Certainly an older baby who has gotten used to sucking on a synthetic nipple over a substantial period of time may well have lost the skill or the inclination to drink directly from the breast. But despite ongoing efforts, there has been no scientific success in proving the existence of 'nipple confusion' after a small number of uses of synthetic nipples. A 1992 study found absolutely no difference in breastfeeding success between young infants who were given a bottle a day in addition to breastfeeding and those who were exclusively breastfed,[39] while a 1997 study found that only 4% of 'lactation failure' could be attributed to some combination of infant frustration and nipple confusion.[40] Many medical researchers now claim not only that threats of nipple confusion have been highly exaggerated but also that these threats terrorize mothers, and in turn the fear instilled by the possibility of using bottles makes breastfeeding relationships more stressful and hard to establish.[41] Ruth Lawrence's textbook on breastfeeding for medical professionals admits to a lack of clear scientific verification of the phenomenon of nipple confusion but then recommends discouraging mothers' use of bottles anyhow, because their occasional use can start a "downward spiral" toward the cessation of breastfeeding. This is an ironic conclusion, given that she has just admitted that the evidence we expected for bottles initiating such a downward spiral does *not* exist.[42]

Pacifiers are another kind of displaceable nipple that can stand for the separation of mother and infant. Children with pacifiers in their mouths are portrayed as cyborg monsters of the mother's own making, with displaced body parts that ought to be on the mother's body connected to their mouths. In turn, mothers who use pacifiers are portrayed as lazy, as initiating a lifetime pattern of oral addiction in their children, and as using an artificial substitute for their own bodily labor and availability. Janet Tamaro writes, "What if the person closest to you shoved rubber in your mouth each time you tried to tell him or her that you were having a problem?"[43] La Leche League warns mothers that a pacifier "can never substitute for a mother."[44] *What to Expect the First Year* expands on the thought:

> There is the ever-present temptation to use the pacifier as a convenient substitute for the attention she herself should be providing for her child. The well-meaning mother who offers the pacifier to make sure her baby has adequate sucking experience may soon find herself popping in a pacifier the moment he becomes fussy. . . . She may use it to get the baby off to sleep instead of reading him a story, to ensure quiet when she's on the phone instead of picking him up and consoling him while she's chatting, to buy his silence while she's picking out a pair of new shoes instead of involving him in the interaction . . . each time you consider plugging it in, ask yourself whether it's the pacifier or you the baby needs.[45]

These passages articulate a genuine risk; surely pacifiers have sometimes compromised the quality of mothering in these ways. Still, the rhetoric of this last passage is worth analyzing. The mother 'finds herself' popping in a pacifier—she is a passive victim of temptation rather than an agent who has made choices about her mothering practices. This lazy mother who has given way to temptation engages in a series of highly gendered and trivialized activities—shopping for shoes and chatting (as opposed to perhaps writing or making a business call). Most significantly, what this passage shares with the two shorter ones is the fear that the pacifier will substitute for *the mother herself*—for the whole process of mothering. It seems to me that this fear is underwritten by the substitution of the breast for the mother and mothering that is already in place. The ideology of the Fetish Mother already construes the mother as defined by her proximity to the infant via the breast, and the complex process of mothering as somehow contained in the mute act of suckling. If the mother just is her suckled breast, and mothering just is suckling, then if an infant suckles a displaced, artificial breast such as a pacifier, it stands to reason that the pacifier is substituting for the mother. While the real concern, it seems, should be that babies get adequate attention, stimulation, and complex interaction rather than a quick physical source of comfort, the rhetorical focus of these passages is upon the fear of substituting the displaced nipple for the real maternal body—a substitution that only makes sense once the two are figured as importantly analogous. The rhetorical force of the vilification of pacifiers seems to rest on their status as displaced and artificial breasts/mothers that physically separate the bodies of mother and infant, rather than on an appropriate concern for their possible use as substitutes for complex, interactive attention. (Significantly, mothers who breastfeed their children to provide them with a source of comfort long after the nutritional bene-fits of breast milk have become negligible—which surely involves no great intellectual stimulation of the child or complex engaged labor from the mother—are never portrayed as especially disengaged, lazy, or self-centered.)

EMBODIED MOTHERHOOD

As I mentioned at the start of this chapter, the fetishistic status of the nursing, extended body takes the vast and intricate skills, elaborate embodied involvement, reflective and critical judgment, learning, and grueling and creative commitment that constitute good mothering and reduces them, at least figuratively, to a mute spatial continuity be-tween mother and infant.[46] When proximity and the bond of milk are taken as equivalent to successful mothering, breast milk that is dis-placed from the mother's body becomes somehow a fundamental threat to mothering, and this mythic reasoning shows up even in crit-ically aware academic literature.

In her recent work *At the Breast*, which is a critical examination of breastfeeding practices and ideologies from the point of view of qualitative social science, Linda Blum argues that we should "resist separating the embodied process—the mother with the baby at the breast—from its product, the human milk."[47] She approves of La Leche League for critiquing pumped breast milk as a 'disembodied product' in contrast with the 'reciprocal, relational' process of direct breast-feeding. Blum uses the catch phrase 'embodied motherhood' to refer to motherhood that centrally includes direct breastfeeding, and she praises La Leche League's 'maternalist model' of mothering for giving primacy to 'embodied motherhood' (while gently criticizing this model for being racist and classist in its implementation, although not, according to her, in its essence). Accordingly, Blum argues that breast pumps are alienating devices employed by medical and work-place institutions to rob mothers of an *embodied* relationship to their children. Her chapter on the history and sociology of breast pumps is called "Disembodied Motherhood."

Blum's suggestion that the embodied dimensions of motherhood can be reduced to or even concentrated in the act of direct breastfeed-ing does grave intellectual and ethical injustice to the actual *embod-ied* process of mothering. The practices of mothering, and parenting more generally, are deeply and thoroughly embodied processes no mat-ter what. Nothing as self-standing and with such a specific function as a breast pump could ever possibly 'disembody' mothering. Mothers, whether they breastfeed or not, spend the better part of several years developing and using sensitive and complicated bodily skills and receptive capacities: comforting a newborn, and then an older baby, and then a toddler, and then an older child whose pride in her independence has to be respected; playing with a baby, bathing and dressing her, holding a toddler's hand when she needs comfort and safety but letting go at just the right moment, and so on ad infinitum (and sometimes ad nauseum). For that matter, infant feeding itself is a complexly and essentially embodied practice, however it is accomplished. All parents know that learning to feed a baby—learning the rhythm of his cues as to when and what and how he wants to eat, when to offer food, when to leave him alone, and so forth—is itself a challenging, reciprocal, and highly embodied process, regardless of what he is eating and via what delivery mechanism.

Underlying the notion that breastfeeding is the 'embodiment' of motherhood and that pumping somehow 'disembodies' motherhood is a naïve and anachronistic notion of embodiment. In the heyday of the Enlightenment, philosophers and scientists generally contrasted 'bodies' with 'minds' or 'spirits.' Impressed by the birth of Newtonian physics, and reacting against Aristotelian functionalism, Enlightenment thinkers often conceived of bodies as properly possessing only those nonintentional, mechanical properties that were recognized as efficacious within this new physics, such as size, mass, and shape. This picture, which uses a specific kind of object of physics as the primary model of material bodies in general, requires us to posit some immaterial animator in order to make up for having reduced the body itself to brute, mute matter with no inherent principles of animation.[48] But twentieth-century philosophers reconceived human activity as the work of the body itself rather than as some immaterial infusion into it. The human body is not a static object devoid of meaning, along the model of the traditional Newtonian object of physics, but a being that in its very materiality is engaged in projects, directed toward the world, receptive in specific ways to its surroundings, and involved in complicated reciprocal relations with other bodies.[49] For something to be *embodied*, then, is not for it to be reducible to some kind of mute, nonintentional physicality. On the contrary, the hallmark of an *embodied* practice is that it involves the body itself in complex, directed, sensitive behavior. To have an embodied relationship with someone (or something) is *not* just to be next to it, or up against it. One can do this without involving what is distinctive about the human body at all. Rather, an embodied relationship with something is one that intertwines the material projects and agency of the body with that object, at the level of concrete practice.[50]

I doubt that we can coherently compare 'how embodied' activities are, although we can look at the differing extents to which these activities draw upon the capacities and potentialities of our bodies. As such, breastfeeding seems far from having earned any special status amidst mothering practices, to say the least. Any central practice of mothering—teaching, comforting, feeding, dressing, singing—is essentially embodied. Notice that we cannot be successful at any of these tasks by thinking them through and deciding how to proceed intellectually. Our bodies must learn, in a great amount of detail, how to respond appropriately and respectfully and helpfully to the bodies of our children. In contrast, breastfeeding, once it is well established, is a fairly straightforward physical act and does little to draw upon our distinctive bodily capacities and skills.

The reduction of motherhood to an embodied relation, and the reduction of this embodied relation to one of proximity, misrepresents not just metaphysical but ethical and political reality. The American Academy of Pediatrics claims that through breastfeeding, the infant "will come to understand that even as his world expands he can continue to count on you for physical comfort and emotional support."[51] It is hard to avoid reading this as suggesting that without breastfeeding, children will not come to count on their mothers in the same way. This prediction is grounded in the elevation of breastfeeding to the privileged essence of the whole embodied process of physically and emotionally supporting an infant—or perhaps it insinuates that non-breastfeeding mothers will for some reason be remiss in the much larger and more complicated project of providing this support. At least as troubling is the implication here that a mother who places her breast in her child's mouth has *thereby* done what it takes to physically and emotionally support her child. Similarly, Janet Tamaro writes that "breastfeeding *represents* a style of parenting: right off the bat you're willing to adjust your life to your baby's and give him a lot of love."[52] Again, we smell the suggestion that activities other than breastfeeding don't require this adjustment, or that non-breastfeeding mothers would for some reason be less likely or able to make these adjustments and give this love. Tamaro's use of the term 'represent' here is slippery—I take it that she means that breastfeeding *manifests* this style of parenting and doesn't just symbolize it, but the language of representation does reveal some of the emblematic and mythic status that breastfeeding has taken on. Both these passages erase the embodied labor of engaged mothers, whether or not they breastfeed, and fetishize and inflate the power of the proximity of the breast at the cost of portraying the true strenuous demands of motherhood.

Not surprisingly, the synecdochal substitution of breastfeeding for good, embodied mothering is complemented by a metonymic association between bottle feeding and uncaring, disembodied mothering. Indeed, as Jules Law points out, formula feeding is often taken as a symbol and a summation of mother-infant separation.[53] In a remarkably histrionic passage (in an altogether irresponsible essay replete with undocumented misinformation) Kathleen Weir writes, "Mothers who bottle feed may not understand that a large element of an infant's eating is the physicality of being held and reassured by the mother's eyes and sounds. Contrast that experience with being left in a cold, dark room, in a wooden cage, with a bottle propped up on a blanket, and it is easy to understand the decay of Western culture."[54] Here, Weir directly associates bottle feeding itself with the abandonment of *any* physical relationship between the mother and the child—the total alienation of the maternal body from the scene of the infant. Making a similar point about a different text, Law points out that "throughout their book, Jelliffe and Jelliffe associatively and insidiously move back and forth between 'artificial feeding' and 'early separation,' the latter defined either elastically or not at all. The overall implication is that formula feeding is scientifically equivalent to a mother's abandoning of her infant, with potentially catastrophic results."[55] In our imagination of both the benefits of breastfeeding and the risks of bottle feeding, the physical mechanics of the feeding relationship have become iconic substitutes for the entire mothering relationship.

Ironically, Linda Blum accuses the pumping process of 'fetishizing' mothers' *milk*, by allowing the milk to stand in for the entire mother.[56] It is quite striking that she doesn't notice that pumping could *only* be seen as effecting such a substitution once we *already* fetishize the feeding process and take the bond of milk as encapsulating the whole of motherhood. If we take breast milk as a symbolic stand-in for the whole of mothering, then we may well 'read' milk that has been mechanically displaced from the breast as a further, alienated stand-in. But if we remain critically aware of how a history of symbolic and concrete ideological practices has reduced the vast and multidimensional project of motherhood to the breast-mouth relation and the transference of milk that it involves, then we will not be tempted to interpret this inarticulate milk—displaced or not—as in any way equivalent to the mother herself. It is remarkable that a critical scholar such as Blum could not notice the ideology behind her sense that the act of moving the feeding process a few inches away from the mother's breast could 'disembody' her or alienate her from the body of her infant.

DENATURING THE BREAST

In fact, overwhelming numbers of North American women who feed their children breast milk rely on pumps at least to some extent. Given the realities of women's jobs and lives, most mothers have to take extraordinary measures if they are to continue nursing a baby without pumping at least some milk. I have not managed to find any statistics on what percentage of breastfeeding mothers use a pump at some point—an absence in the literature that is itself significant—but it is clearly a large percentage. Furthermore, there is no scientific evidence that there are *any* benefits to infants from drinking breast milk directly from the breast as opposed to from a bottle, assuming basic sanitation conditions are met; even the psychological benefits of breast milk seem to accrue independent of the delivery mechanism, as far as we know.[57]

Given what an enormous advance the modern breast pump is as a means for enabling women to offer breast milk to their children, when their life circumstances and choices would otherwise preclude their doing so, one would hope and even expect that public health institutions would be huge boosters of breast pumps as important mainstream tools in infant feeding. Indeed, empirical research shows that one of the most effective ways of getting women to continue breastfeeding is to support and encourage the use of breast pumps. In one recent study, for instance, interventions that supported pumping raised the rate of working mothers still breastfeeding at six months from 6% to 53%.[58]

But in fact, pumping and express feeding is positioned by a wide majority of health sources as an inherently marginal and suboptimal feeding practice. Lauwers and Woessner's 500-page 1990 textbook, *Counseling the Nursing Mother*, mentions pumping only in a single section of a few pages near the end, as a subheading within a chapter called 'Special Aids and Techniques.' The authors introduce this section with the claim that "In the course of her breastfeeding experience, a mother does not usually require any *special gadgets or breastfeeding aids*."[59] They thereby mark pumping as an exceptional and artificial practice as opposed to a normal and important part of feeding breast milk to infants. The La Leche League guide discusses pumping briefly in a chapter called "Common Concerns." They introduce the topic of pumps with the comment, "Experience has taught us that breastfeeding proceeds most smoothly when kept as simple and natural as possible. But there are some circumstances in which a product designed to aid breastfeeding can be helpful."[60] This text portrays the mother who pumps as a downtrodden hero, conquering adversity in order to get breast milk to her child, but it never questions (or supports) the presumption that direct breastfeeding is the superior feeding practice. Perhaps most tellingly, the American Academy of Pediatrics asks mothers to "remind" their husbands that "expressed milk fed with a bottle is a welcome but less desirable substitute for the *real thing*,"[61] although it offers no evidence or explanation for this lesser status.

Pumped milk is figured as unsanitary and polluted in comparison to directly delivered milk. New mothers who 'must' pump are given highly hyperbolic information about what is needed in order to keep their milk safe. Doctors and advice manuals tell women not to leave breast milk unrefrigerated for over an hour, and also that every bit of the pump and bottles must be sterilized with boiling water or a professional sterilizer for the first four months of an infant's life. In fact breast milk stays fresh for six hours at room temperature,[62] and of course the skin of a nursing mother does not even approximate this level of sterility; milk can remain on her breast and later enter an infant's mouth for hours or even days. (Breastfeeding mothers are in fact counseled against using any soap on their breasts for fear of upsetting the 'natural' balance of the skin.)[63] At the same time, the vast percentage of the (relatively few) scientific studies that concern expressed breast milk focus on its potential contamination.[64] In these ways, pumped milk is implicitly and explicitly positioned as a degraded and dangerous substance. This is not surprising, in ideological context— once the maternal body has been rent asunder and its milk displaced, it becomes once again an unruly, hysterical body with the power to contaminate and corrupt, rather than an emblem of natural order. In fact, these concerns over the pollution of pumped milk are neat rhetorical replacements for the analogous concerns about the pollution from the breast of the wet nurse or the wayward mother during the preceding couple of centuries.

Virtually all of the scientific and lay literature on infant feeding simply divides the feeding possibilities into two, namely 'breast' vs. 'bottle' feeding, where this very division elides the distinction between the means of delivery and the substance fed. Generally 'bottle feeding' is taken to mean formula feeding, and 'breast feeding' is taken to mean direct breastfeeding, in which case feeding expressed milk doesn't even show up as a possibility—but sometimes it is simply unclear or indeterminate how the breast/bottle distinction is being used. This invisibility and lack of clarity is common to scientific and lay literature alike. For example, in the "101 reasons to breastfeed" listed by the breastfeeding advocacy group Promom, reason #50 is that "breast milk is always the right temperature."[65] And Katherine Dettwyler claims that "today, few people would argue that formula/bottle feeding is superior, or even equivalent, to breastfeeding."[66] Indeed she suggests that "bottle fed" children should be charged higher premiums for health coverage.[67] This suggestion conflates the *method of delivery* with the *substance delivered* (not to mention being politically problematic, given the lower breastfeeding rates among low-income women whose workplaces are less likely to allow the time, space, and support for ongoing lactation).

Scientific studies frequently build the binary opposition between 'breast' and 'bottle' feeding, and the corresponding elision between feeding substance and delivery method, into their titles and their methodologies. To give just one example, a recent study asked women how they intended to feed their children: breast, bottle, or breast and bottle. This question literally needs to be taken as asking about delivery method, but presumably respondents interpreted it to some (imprecise) degree as asking about substance fed as well.[68] Scientific studies of infant feeding not only re-entrench the breast/bottle dichotomy but also usually show no recognition that the distinction between substance and delivery might matter to the methodology of their studies and the interpretation of their results.

The systematic opposition between 'breast' and 'bottle,' the elision between substance and delivery method, and the silencing of pumping as a possibility all help make it difficult for mothers to find and correctly interpret the medical facts about the feeding choices available to them. Still, many women do end up using pumped breast milk as the primary or the exclusive food for their infants, which is not something that is easy to tell from any published sources, but which becomes clear from perusing chat rooms and trading anecdotes with friends. Women find their own way to this feeding option, but they do so without the benefit of much clear medical information or institutional guidance or support. My point here is not to serve as an advocate for the specific practice of exclusive or primary expressed milk feeding, although I am convinced that if cultural rhetoric were different, many more women would see this as a very attractive feeding option. (It clearly has all the medical benefits of direct breastfeeding, and at the same time enables mothers to work and pursue activities that involve more than trivial separations from their infants, and enables other people in a mother's circle of potential caregivers to fully participate in feeding.) My reason for focusing on this practice is rather to highlight how the dichotomous spatial logic of proximity and separation has concretely and pervasively governed our thought about infant feeding so that anything other than direct breastfeeding is understood as an artificial interruption in the extended maternal body.

Expectant and new mothers are inundated with romanticized visions of the nursing body and dire warnings about the risks of failing to breastfeed, by health professionals, community groups, and the culture at large, while at the very same time almost no institutional practices are in place for getting breast milk to infants when the mother's breast as a direct delivery mechanism is not available for whatever reason. Human milk banks are rare and the means of access to them are obscure, communal breastfeeding is socially taboo, and pumping itself is underemphasized and denigrated in practice. In other words, there is an important mismatch between our cultural, rhetorical valuation of breastfeeding as a symbol of proper maternity and our pragmatic commitment to the project of getting breast milk to infants. We are apparently loyal to breast milk's original delivery mechanism—the mother's lactating breast—far more than to the public health goal of getting the milk itself to infants, delivered by whatever means.

THE MYTH OF THE INFINITELY BOUNTIFUL BREAST AND ITS MAGIC MILK

In our post-Enlightenment culture, we use a mythical logic for imagining breast milk itself; its evil twin, formula; and the mother's milk-producing body. The body of the Fetish Mother is figured as a magical space—one whose special powers of production and provision break the laws of conservation. This body can provide for its children on demand, at no cost to itself—it gives without losing anything. This myth of the infinitely bountiful breast was central to the Republican symbolism of the natural body politic, and it now inflects our medical, political, and economic understanding of infant feeding. We treat breastfeeding as 'cost free,' in contrast to formula: "Human milk is the ultimate in renewable resources," proclaims one article archived by La Leche League,[69] and "Breast milk is free," according to Promom's list of '101 reasons to breastfeed.'[70] In the face of such cost-free bounty, it seems, only ignorance or selfishness could keep a mother from breastfeeding. In reality, however, breastfeeding exacts a huge toll on a mother's body and uses up resources that must be constantly replenished. When underfed women nurse, their own bones end up donating calcium, and their blood donates iron.[71] Women with limited reserves are thus put at substantial risk by breastfeeding, although this risk has received virtually no scientific attention as a public health issue, for instance as an issue of special concern in the developing world, where attention has focused almost entirely on the dangers of formula.[72]

The Fetish Mother, as she appears in our cultural imagination, is immune to the logic of conservation. After all, the pure, ideal maternal body can nourish an entire nation. La Republique, who sustains and replenishes a nation through her breasts, never needs to scarf down calories and carbohydrates as her blood sugar crashes, nor does she collapse with exhaustion with bags under her eyes. She remains unchanged as her breast provides without end, her body a space that can expand indefinitely. The breasts of the Fetish Mother are often figured as food—peaches, melons, apples, ice cream—which can be consumed without any cost to the body that bears it. Eva Marie Simms writes that during breastfeeding, she "felt heavy and complacent, bovine and earthy, content to empty [her]self out in an *infinite stream*."[73] We are so used to seeing the nursing maternal body represented as undepletable that we are jarred and disturbed by Scott Brooks' recent painting "Fortitude" (figure 5.1), in which a drained and exhausted mother's life force and reserves appear siphoned off to her breast, upon which her infant possessively places his mouth and arm.

Parenting manuals regularly remind mothers that insufficient milk supplies virtually never occur 'naturally.' Mothers are advised to stand strong and have faith in their own bounty rather than cave into the temptation to interrupt their natural, extended bodies with instruments of artificial separation such as bottles and pumps. Breastfeeding and mothering manuals contain numerous inspirational anecdotes about mothers who fed twins or triplets exclusively with their own breasts. The manuals abound with a double message. On the one hand, portray the ideal maternal body as capable of unlimited feats of production, telling mothers that "your breasts are never empty." This is technically true, because milk is produced as it is expressed, but misleading because it suggests unending bounty and fullness when in fact a breast may be exhausted to the point of only being able to produce a

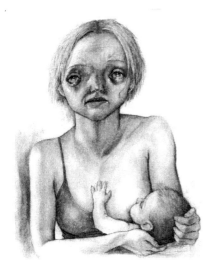

Figure 5.1. Scott Brooks, *Fortitude*, from the series *The Virtues*, 2002. Privately owned; reprinted courtesy of the artist.

tiny drop at a time. On the other hand, they suggest that insufficient milk is the fault of the imperfect mother who interrupts the workings of her natural body. Mothers are told that milk supply is indefatigably keyed to demand, as long as 'artificial' interruptions of the extended nursing body are not introduced; any violations of the harmonious fit between supply and demand are thus the fault of the mother who doesn't follow the natural order. They are warned that supplementing with formula, being separated from the baby and missing a feeding, and creating 'nipple confusion' by letting the child suck on an artificial nipple are all maternal causes of diminished milk supply.[74]

Given all this, it is interesting to note that not having enough milk is the single most common reason that women give for ceasing to breastfeed earlier than they had originally intended.[75] Since it is indeed quite rare for a woman to be unable to produce sufficient milk for her baby, we need to ask why so many women perceive themselves as unable to do so, and we also need to worry about how many women, when they believe this (rightly or wrongly), quit breastfeeding altogether rather than supplement with formula or expressing extra milk. I suggest that women may be intimidated by the high standards set by the infinitely bountiful breast of the Fetish Mother and underconfident in the face of her serene 'natural' productivity. We are encouraged, during pregnancy, to think of our soon-to-be lactating bodies in rapturous, magical terms. When we encounter the reality of our very unmagical bodies—exhausted, leaky, sometimes incapable of letdown, sometimes absent, sometimes not up to the task of meeting our newborn's needs, sometimes experiencing pain and irritation rather than ecstatic unity during breastfeeding—it is no surprise that we cease to identify with the Fetish Mother and suspect ourselves of instead being unruly and untrustworthy.

It is not only the body of the lactating mother to which we attribute a magical logic but also the milk itself, insofar as it comes directly as a gift from the proximate breast.[76] In *So That's What They're For: Breastfeeding Basics*, Janet Tamaro reprints a paragraph-long list of the ingredients of an infant formula. She contrasts this with breast milk, which is supposed to be 'simple,' where this simplicity itself apparently functions as direct support for its superiority.[77] The length of the ingredient list is presumably supposed to testify to the 'unnatural' status of formula. But of course, breast milk itself has an incredibly complex composition, and it is this very complexity, in part, that has made it so difficult to replicate its quality—its composition is perhaps intractably elaborate. The force of Tamaro's point cannot rationally rest on an inference from number of ingredients to inferior worth but rather stems from the fetishized status of the milk from the mother's breast as *essentially* simple or unitary. Its many components don't count against it because they are 'naturally' unified. In this way, much like the extended nursing body itself, breast milk functions as a symbolic microcosm of well-ordered nature.

While breast milk is portrayed as a substance that is inherently natural, orderly, and harmony-producing, formula is portrayed as having almost magically corrupting powers. "Formula for Disaster" reads the title of one electronic article for mothers, and one subsection is titled, "Are formula-fed babies at risk to be both poisoned and dumber?" The article is fronted by a picture of a monstrous, cyborg breast with an artificial bottle nipple in place of a human nipple.[78] La Leche League writes in their guide, "Does one bottle of formula make that much difference? We wish we could say that it doesn't, but we can't. Even one bottle of formula can be a problem for some babies because of allergies. Animal studies have also shown that introducing formula may upset the balance of enzymes and nutrients in the digestive system and interfere with the protective qualities your milk provides."[79] The idea that artificial bottles and milk can do instant harm by upsetting delicate natural balances plays upon the privileging of breastfeeding as a preservation of a 'natural order' that has normative force. Mothers' milk is a harmonious and well-ordering substance, while formula is a disordering agent that threatens to disrupt and corrupt this natural balance.

The status of breast milk as an essentially well-ordered substance is further underscored by the occasional portrayal of cows' milk as a monstrous food for human infants. Literature on infant feeding often points out that human milk is 'for humans' while cows milk is 'for cows,' and by implication somehow inherently *not* for humans. According to one breastfeeding advocacy website, "the fact that human beings can even drink the milk of another species is sort of amazing when you stop to think about it."[80] This is an extraordinary claim given that humans are omnivores and consume other animals' products on a regular basis; the specific uncanniness that is attributed to other animals' *milk* here rides on the special fetishized status of breast milk and its 'naturalness,' and not on any inherent problem with cross-species consumption. The human child drinking the milk of a beast is figured as a monstrous hybrid, in contrast with the well-ordered natural nursling. Of course, human milk does have all sorts of benefits for human infants that cows' milk doesn't have, but the simple fact of the bestial source of cows' milk has no empirical import.[81]

We are all familiar with the litany of threats levied against mothers that substitute bottle-fed infant formula for the gifts of the proximate breast. They are told they are putting their children at risk of allergies, compromised resistance to disease, obesity, diabetes, arthritis, constipation, lower IQ, compromised self-esteem, antisocial behavior, ear and respiratory tract infections, speech disorders, and much more. Very few experts would claim that all of these supposed risks have been carefully substantiated. While it is unquestionable that breast milk is a healthier primary food for infants than is formula, there are reasons to think that we need to take our cultural fear of bottle feeding, and of the breach it makes in the extended body of the Fetish Mother, as problematically ideological and not just as a rational response to new medical knowledge. While to some extent this list is a product of our latest medical discoveries, we need to be attuned to the ways in which formula functions mythologically as a source of corruption, in ways that outstrip scientific reason.

For example, anthropologist and renowned breastfeeding specialist Katherine Dettwyler fantasizes about a day when all formula carries a surgeon general's warning that includes the claim that "the use of infant formula is known to *reduce* children's IQ as much as lead poisoning does, and *hinders* the strong affective bonds between mother and child."[82] It is clear, upon reflection, that the claim that formula 'reduces' IQ is incoherent, as it presupposes that the infant had some fixed, higher IQ in place before formula came along and corrupted it. There is no scientific support for any such claim, nor is there any meaningful extension of the notion of IQ to neonates. There is no concrete scientific support for the idea that formula feeding results in lower maternal bonds, and especially not for the dubiously coherent idea that it *gets in the way* of their (presumably natural) development. The idea that formula 'hinders' the bond between mother and child or 'lowers' IQ implies an originary breastfed infant, already there in potential and then deformed by formula. We see here an implicit model, which is ideologically powerful but scientifically meaningless, in which the infant is a natural object with a determinate potential character whether or not that character is ever actualized, into which formula is a corrupting, unnatural intervention—a foreign poison, like lead, and a force that rends open the naturally bonded bodies of mother and child.

We need to remember that the social panic over the mere spatial separation of the mother's and infant's bodies during feeding substantially predates current medical discoveries concerning the advantages of breast milk, and indeed it predates the existence of commercial formula. Rhetorically speaking, the suspicion and demonization of formula can be read as a pretty straightforward transmutation of the cultural suspicion and demonization of wet-nursing in the wake of Rousseau and the Revolution. As we saw, post-Rousseauians thought the displacement of the maternal body from the site of feeding was 'unnatural,' and most of the same charges that are now levied against formula-fed infants—general weakness of constitution, psychological damage, proneness to disease, stupidity, and so forth—were levied against wet-nursed children. My point is that the normative *naturalization* of the proximity between breast and mouth predates any particular concerns about *unnatural* milk substitutes. Likewise, our separation anxieties supersede the body of medical knowledge that might support these anxieties in any particular era.[83]

Here and elsewhere, what is important to notice, for my purposes, is not that the various recommendations and pressures on maternal bodies are false or misguided from the point of view of the concrete benefits to children's health and well-being. Rather, I am trying to focus on how these recommendations are packaged, which is as ways of normatively enforcing a figure of a unique 'natural' mother and her extended body with its nonfungible special power to nurture its own infant—a power whose uniqueness seems to be taken as too primitive to require scientific examination. The spatial bond between mother and infant serves as a mythological and overdetermined locus of our lost nostalgic history, of nature, of virtue, of health, and of proper mothering. This extended body has a public place and significance that far outstrips any particular, concrete empirical claims that can be made about it.

THE LACTATING BODY AS SCIENTIFIC OBJECT

Systematic scientific studies of the benefits of mother-infant proximity and the dangers of separation are scant.[84] Many of the key figures and movements whose promotion of proximity has captured public attention (such as La Leche League, William and Martha Sears and the attachment theorists, and the object relations theorists) are not interested in engaging in or citing such research, relying instead on anecdotal evidence and interpretations of case studies. References to the 'special closeness,' 'oneness,' and 'unique bond' enabled by direct breastfeeding often form the rhetorical packaging for scientific studies, even while they rarely constitute their substance or topic. Even within scientific communities, the specific connection between direct breast-feeding and bonding generally seems to be taken as so self-evident as to be immune from the need for scientific study.[85]

To the extent that there has been or can be scientific work in this area, we need to treat it with some care.[86] It is hard to know how one would go about giving operational definitions of 'special closeness' or 'oneness,' or even 'bonding.' Indeed, the 'bond' that is supposedly established through proximity, along with its purported powers to found psychic, moral, and civic health, is itself such an amorphous relationship that it is not clear how we could identify its presence or absence, *except* through the question-begging employment of figures of the spatially extended maternal body. For example, scientific studies often build the elision between breast-mouth proximity and the entire human relationship between mother and infant into their methodology. Thus for instance, in "Kangaroo Mother Care and the Bonding Hypothesis,"[87] the authors use breastfeeding 'success,' defined in terms of duration, as a *measure* of successful attachment.[88]

In a similar question-begging move, many studies that examine the relationship between breastfeeding and psychological health or developmental benefits fail to control for other dimensions of parenting style and parent-child relations, including amount of other kinds of tactile contact, thereby presuming that breastfeeding can stand in for all of these forms of mother-child interaction.[89] This is a methodologically crucial omission, especially in a culture where (a) there is enough pressure to associate breastfeeding with 'good' mothering that mothers who do not breastfeed may well *on average* be less concerned or engaged with their infants in other ways (since after all, social pressure wouldn't count as pressure if it didn't influence behavior), and (b) bottle-feeding mothers are disproportionately low-income working mothers who for various reasons, including inflexible work situations and long hours, may be in less of a position to engage in ideal parenting. Before any claims can be made about the psychic or developmental benefits of breastfeeding, studies would need to compare breastfed and non-breastfed children while systematically controlling for the amount and forms of other kinds of contact, for parenting style, and for the caregivers' overall involvement in caretaking. We cannot *assume* that for the purposes of a study, breastfeeding can serve as a stand-in for involved, high-contact parenting, nor can we assume that dimensions of parenting other than feeding are not significant factors in need of experimental control in bonding and psychic development studies.

In another variation on the theme of the methodological elision of breastfeeding, proximity, and good mothering as a whole, Katherine Dettwyler interprets results showing a correlation between *tactile contact* and psychic health as *directly* supporting a strong causal connection between *breastfeeding* and psychic health. Dettwyler claims that the "the tactile, olfactory, visual and gustatory interactions that take place between mother and child during breastfeeding" are "*required* for the *proper* physical, cognitive and emotional development of the child."[90] In order to support this exceptionally strong claim, which rules out even the *possibility* that a bottle-fed child could develop 'properly,' Dettwyler cites Harry Harlow's famous experiments, which demonstrated that infant rhesus monkeys preferred cloth "mothers" with no milk to wire "mothers" with milk—that is, that they preferred tactile contact with a nonlactating, soft nonmaternal body to a milk-providing, hard nonmaternal body. To take this as evidence for the essential benefits of direct breastfeeding requires the deep presumption that the *whole* tactile and sensory interaction between mother and child occurs during the breastfeeding process (or is somehow summed up and encapsulated in that process). Without this reductionist assumption, Harlow's results if anything give prima facie support to the *opposite* of Dettwyler's conclusion: they suggest that the milk delivery process is *less* important to proper development than other sorts of tactile interaction, which certainly do not require a lactating maternal body. If Dettwyler's figuration of the nursing body did not lead her to assume that a non-breastfeeding mother is one that is overall less able to physically meet its child's psychic needs, then she could not use this result to support the specific importance of breastfeeding to good mothering, and hence her argument is directly circular. Furthermore, Dettwyler uncritically accepts Harlow's rhetorically loaded use of the term 'mothers' to refer to the cloth and wire dummies, thereby accepting that mothering can be crystallized in a single dimension of proximate contact.[91]

Most informational literature that promotes breastfeeding—which includes almost all the literature available for contemporary pregnant women and new mothers—is guilty of a rhetorical slide from the medical evidence supporting the benefits of breast milk as an infant food to the glorification of a romanticized vision of the actual act of breastfeeding, with little or no marking of where medical advice leaves off and ideological images of appropriate bonding begin. For example, the American Academy of Pediatrics, in its official guide to breastfeeding, moves smoothly from a concrete discussion of the empirically documented immunological and nutritional benefits of breast milk to the unverifiable claim that "your newborn also benefits from the physical closeness of nursing. Thrust from the close, dark womb into an overwhelming experience of bright lights, loud noises, and new smells, your baby needs the reassurance of your continued physical presence. By holding him safe in your arms and nourishing him from your body, you offer him a sense of continuity from pre- to post-birth life."[92] The inherently authoritative position of this work masks the unsupported and imprecise nature of this claim—a claim that once again models the mother-child relationship on the material continuity of pregnancy.

This AAP guide freely interjects inspirational messages in a first-person voice, which may or may not be actual quotations, into the text: "We are so in tune with each other, thanks to the bonding of breastfeeding—and I can see that this will make other areas of parenting, such as discipline, easier," opines "Elise," and "Jennifer" attributes a rather implausible grasp of abstract symbolism to her seven-month-old when she informs us that "every time Maddie is hungry and I offer her the breast, I am showing her in a really basic way that I'm here when it counts and her needs will be met. Even when I'm at work and she gets breast milk from a cup, I think she gets the message that she can depend on Mom for the important things."[93]

My main discomfort is not with these rosy rhetorical flourishes and 'opinions' in and of themselves, although they strike me as nearly vacuous regurgitations of ideologically packaged sentiments. Rather, I am disturbed by the significance of the context in which they appear. Wearing the firmly anchored mantle of medical and scientific authority, the American Academy of Pediatrics makes no effort to separate this type of (pseudo) testimony from the medical facts that they, as an organization, are in a position to authoritatively convey. This kind of slide is dangerous, both because it fails to mark for women where fact leaves off and ideology begins, and also because it suggests to women who do not experience ecstatic union with their infants during breast-feeding, or who have trouble establishing successful breastfeeding for whatever reason, that they have failed their children in the eyes of the medical establishment. They may even believe that there is no point trying to get breast milk to their infants by other means, such as pumps, since they have already failed at the 'breastfeeding experience.'[94]

THE REEMERGENCE OF THE UNRULY MOTHER

I have been focusing in this chapter on the cultural and medical glorification of direct breastfeeding and the corresponding demonization and fear of bottles and formula. As we saw in chapter 3, however, even as we glorify the nursing body of the Fetish Mother, we often deem many actual mothers' bodies as measuring poorly against this ideal and treat their milk as requiring regulation or even replacement with artificial substitutes. At the moment, our culture has a quite inclusive view of whose breasts get to count as able to work their proximate magic. We saw in chapter 3 that at the end of the nineteenth century, when infant formula first became a major industry, messages about the superiority of breastfeeding *for proper mothers with proper bodies* were paired with messages about the various ways in which maternal bodies could be inadequate and in need of medical surveillance and intervention, and in these cases breastfeeding was often discouraged. During the mid-twentieth century, the pendulum swung even farther in that direction: formula feeding was 'in vogue' and vigorously promoted by medical and community institutions. Breastfeeding was often seen as slightly distasteful and primitive, even bestial, in comparison with the clean scientific precision of formula.[95] For those raised or mothering at this time, the current swing toward breastfeeding may itself seem a relatively exceptional phenomenon, which would undermine my claim that it represents and participates in an ideology with a deep and pervasive history and force in our culture.

This perspective is undercut somewhat when we take a longer view of history. Pam Carter, for instance, does an excellent job of showing how, over the course of the last couple hundred years, the mid-twentieth-century denigration of breastfeeding and glorification of bottles was actually the exception to the general pro-breastfeeding rule[96] (albeit one that was formative for today's baby boomers and older generation). Indeed, mainstream American public health information for mothers in the 1920s and 1930s not only promoted breastfeeding as the superior choice but also drew upon rhetoric and reasoning very similar to that found in contemporary literature; mothers were told that breast milk boosted the child's immune system, was naturally suited to the child's needs, helped prevent disease, and so on.[97] Breastfeeding was also cast as the more natural, the self-evidently more appropriate, and the more virtuous choice—indeed, a "duty and a privilege" of mothers[98]—while artificial feeding was cast as dangerous. A 1932 state-produced guide tells us, "From all standpoints, maternal nursing, under normal conditions, is the most satisfactory method of nourishing a baby. . . . There is no entirely adequate substitute for satisfactory maternal nursing, and any other food that is given to the young baby is at best a makeshift."[99] And a 1923 guide writes, "There is no question whatever that, generally speaking, the best food for the baby is the milk of its own mother. Anything else, any mixture of other milk or milk products, is at best a second-rate substitute, and always increases the dangers through which the baby must pass to reach early childhood. . . . A *moment's thought* will convince anyone that it is less risky to feed the baby in a natural manner than in any other way. . . . Statistics are at hand in every country to prove that the sickness and death among bottle-fed babies is much greater than among those who are nursed by their mothers."[100]

But rather than focus on the constancies in pro-breastfeeding ideology, I think it is more interesting to consider how the specifics of *both* the pro- and anti-breastfeeding movements have disclosed the highly complex relationship between the ideological life of an ideal, fetishized maternal body and the concrete practices and rhetoric surrounding actual mothers' bodies. Although in coarse terms, mid-twentieth-century attitudes toward the lactating maternal body may appear opposite to our current attitudes as I am portraying them, I think a closer look shows a continuity of concerns. For my claim all along has been that the Fetish Mother and the Unruly Mother exist side by side and complement and constitute one another. Faith in the 'natural' lactating maternal body, as a symbol and source of unity and virtue, is faith in the Fetish Mother, and as we saw in earlier chapters, this never simply translates directly into faith in actual, imperfect mothers' bodies. The 1923 guide I just cited tells mothers, "It is of course true that every mother cannot nurse her baby, and certain other mothers should not. There are some definite contraindications to breastfeeding. . . . The physician should decide in every case."[101] The obvious natural goodness of breastfeeding applies to ideal, fetishized bodies, not real, unruly maternal bodies, which required policing by medical authorities, who in turn functioned as the official measure of appropriate and inappropriate maternal nature.[102]

Despite the current pro-breastfeeding climate, and the current glorification of the extended maternal body, actual medical practices often still intervene in the establishment of breastfeeding when a mother's body appears to be irregular or unruly. So for example, mothers who have cesarean sections (roughly 30% in North America), or an infection during labor, or any other irregularity during childbirth, despite receiving standard messages about the benefits of breastfeeding, are frequently subject to hospital practices that tend to thwart the establishment of breastfeeding. For instance, healthy children are often taken to the NICU after a mother has been given antibiotics, as a 'precaution,' or given bottles in the nursery if their mother has had a c-section. Advice literature and videos about breastfeeding often 'warn' women with non-normative shapes (obese women, small- and large-breasted women) that they may well encounter special difficulties in breastfeeding. Hence at the same time as the Fetish Mother is glorified, and women are strongly encouraged to feel that they fall short as mothers and citizens and women if they don't embody her, it seems that medical and cultural institutions are still fairly quick to treat real mothers as unruly and defective, and *in concrete practice* mothers are often discouraged from breastfeeding as soon as their bodies display 'unnatural' imperfections that defetishize them.[103]

Even at the peak of the formula trend, amidst the heightened quantification, surveillance, and control of birth and early mothering,

the Fetish Mother still occupied a privileged and founding role in our
maternal imagination. Indeed, many of the proximity-based parenting
theories I explored at the start of this chapter—attachment theory, object relations theory, etc.—had their heyday during the height of anti-
breastfeeding sentiment within popular culture. In this context, we
can see the local, mid-twentieth-century distaste for breastfeeding not
as a whole different ideology but as a manifestation of a moment
where for a complex, local cluster of cultural reasons, women's bodies
were more quickly and immediately placed on the side of the unruly,
while the Fetish Mother had a more distanced and mediated relationship to the daily practices and concrete treatment of individual maternal bodies than usual.

The cultural glorification of breastfeeding is not primarily founded
in an appreciation of its concrete medical benefits but in the logic of a
fetish ideal, which will always exist at some distance from mundane
mothers' bodies and exercise normative force over them. Mothers may
be disciplined using this ideal, they may experience guilt at falling
short of it, or they may constitute their expectations and experiences
of their own early motherhood in terms of it, but it is never simply descriptive. Hence it is no surprise that at different eras, the pressure to
conform to this ideal and the fear that the body is unruly and in need
of regulation, quantification, and intervention will play off one another in different proportions and with somewhat different effects.
Given the ongoing dialectic between the figures of the Fetish and Unruly Mother, it should not surprise us that in the mid-twentieth-
century era, when our imaginations were captured by the revolution
in convenience technology, and feminine domestic space was being ordered, homogenized, and sanitized on multiple fronts—by the invention of new gadgets, the onslaught of suburban development, birth
control, and more—we were vastly quicker to judge the mother's body
unruly enough to fall short of the fetish ideal and to require public and
artificial intervention and regulation.[104]

Advertising for infant formula in First World countries has never
tried to claim that the product was essentially better than breast milk
but rather has focused on how mothers' bodies could fail to be up to
the task of breastfeeding, for various reasons real and imagined. This
approach to formula promotion began in the late nineteenth century,
as we saw, and has been employed consistently ever since. In the middle of the twentieth century, when formula feeding was most popular,
a whole host of ways that mothers' bodies could be relevantly unruly
captured the cultural imagination—we worried about insufficient
milk, about milk that was 'toxic' or indigestible to the infant, about
mothers whose own health wasn't up to the rigors of breastfeeding,

and so on.[105] In contrast, formula was presented as a dependable, controlled substance with the sanitized stamp of scientific authority—one that could be minutely quantified in terms of both its contents and how much the child was ingesting, and hence which made a safe and surveyable substitute for the vagaries of the maternal body. Contemporary formula advertisements, which are required by law to state that breastfeeding is the best method of infant feeding, claim that when mothers "can't" breastfeed, their product is the best alternative and the one that most closely simulates proper breast milk.

It is common, in both the scholarly and the advocacy literature on breastfeeding, to make reference to the 'medicalization of pregnancy and motherhood,' a phenomenon that supposedly pushes mothers to bottle feed rather than breastfeed. As Pam Carter points out, such literature is often quick to blame formula companies and a supposedly callous, impersonal, and oppressive medical establishment for women's 'failure' to breastfeed.[106] My sense is that this picture of cultural and medical institutions is much too simple, although some of the insidious and morally unforgivable marketing practices of formula companies should not be understated. In reality, the scientific and medical culture surrounding pregnancy seems all too ready to uncritically reiterate the ideology of the Fetish Mother, at least when it comes to the socially acceptable bodies of First World women. I have argued that these cultures collude with 'lay' culture in confuting the distinction between the delivery method and the substance of infant feeding and in erasing the need for critical tests of assumptions about the normative value and 'bonding power' of the nursing body. We have seen that over the last two centuries, the maternal body has indeed been brought under the scope of medical authority and become an object of medical regulation and surveillance. But this medical authority has not taken away the power of the figure of the Fetish Mother; indeed this authority is often used to buttress and legitimize this power and to penalize and marginalize mothers' bodies when they do not measure up to the standards set by this figure.

IDEOLOGY AND THE CONSTITUTION OF DESIRE

The ideology of the extended maternal body and the fetishization of proximity constitute a space of possible, appropriate, 'natural' maternal desires and likewise a corresponding space of precluded, problematic, 'unnatural' desires. This metric of desire can be in itself an effective conduit for the ideology it reflects. For example, parenting literature often offers *predictions* about what new mothers will 'naturally' find themselves desiring. La Leche League, in its guide, offers such predictions addressed to the mother in the second person, calling upon her to find herself reflected in them: "Along with whatever else you are doing during the day, *you will want to keep your baby close to you as a matter of course.* . . . Nobody else can take your place. . . . You don't have to be a stay-at-home with a breastfed baby. Baby can go *right along with you* almost anywhere you want to go." And again, "*You won't want to leave your baby any more than you have to because babies need their mother.* . . . A mother finds that when she does leave her baby for that long-awaited 'night out' she worries so much about how the baby is getting along that she doesn't really enjoy the occasion."[107] In these passages, expectant and new mothers are not told what would be good for the baby but rather what they will, of their own accord, 'naturally' feel and know once they are mothering—and what they will feel and know is that proximity is good and appropriate and that separation is unnatural and problematic and that their bodies are uniquely able to sustain their infants. The mother who has 'long-awaited' a night out will in fact be reduced to a state of debilitating worry—she has put herself into an unnatural situation of separation. The rhetoric suggests that if 'you' find that you *do* enjoy your night out, the flaw is in your maternality, not in their parenting suggestions.

The claim that your baby can go along with you 'almost anywhere you want to go' imposes interesting restrictions on what kinds of desires are appropriate for new mothers. Indeed, this guide, like many others, is full of examples of mothers satisfying their desires for mobility by taking their babies to shopping malls, parks, friends' houses, and other gendered leisure spaces. The rhetoric of the claim forecloses the possibilities of mothers even having real desires to go to a classical music concert, a research library, an academic talk, a board meeting, or any of many other spaces inappropriate for babies, in which various kinds of serious, perhaps identity-defining projects and passions might be pursued. Such rhetoric casts mothers' desires that conflict with proximity as inappropriate and unnatural.

Indeed, in both the La Leche League guide and in similar works, appropriate mothers' activities to which one can take along a baby are regularly contrasted, *not* with pursuing a meaningful career or other important passions and projects, but simply with 'material' desires for money and consumer goods (or, as we saw earlier, with trivial desires to 'chat' on the phone or go shoe shopping). For example in *The Paradox of Natural Mothering*, Chris Bobel interviews one self-described "natural mother" who contrasts her practices of proximity with what she calls a "materialist standard." She says, "I think those mothers probably feel they are doing everything right—conserving energy, serving schoolchildren, bringing money into their families. But their babies are not *with* their mothers, and that's not OK." Bobel follows up, "Grace asserts that children are forced *apart* to satisfy their parents' needs for material gain."[108] The space of possible maternal desires is thereby flattened into a duality between selfish desires induced by the unnatural world of money, 'materialism,' and separation (into which energy conservation is here mysteriously assimilated) and appropriately domestic desires conducive to proximity.[109]

Such rhetoric not only sets up social standards for what count as acceptable or possible maternal desires but also in fact *constitutes* maternal desires and thereby positions mothers as collaborators in the perpetration of the ideology it reflects. It is interesting to notice how often women claim that La Leche League helped them to articulate feelings they 'already had' but felt unable to express.[110] This process of transforming inchoate feelings, real or imagined, into words cannot help but give shape and new determinacy to those feelings; the articulated feelings will never in fact be identical to the inchoate ones, even if they give the phenomenological illusion of capturing them perfectly. I think that these moments when we 'discover,' through the help of social discourse, a feeling or attitude or feature of our identity as having 'been there all along' tend to be moments marking the constitutive work of ideology. We are especially open to this kind of ideological constitution when we are struggling to stabilize and articulate our feelings and identity anyhow. We saw in the last chapter how the boundaries and the integrity of the self are especially fragile and available for co-option during periods of radical upheaval in one's lived identity. Under most circumstances, giving birth and becoming a primary caregiver of a newborn is such a period of dramatic transformation.[111] When we are in a vulnerable period of transformation, who and what we are, and what we believe and feel, are dynamic and not well formed. Effective ideological interventions can bring determinacy and articulation to our self-characterizations, and they can make this new determinacy appear as the uncovering of an already given, natural fact about us.[112]

MOTHER-LOVE AND THE POLITICS OF PROXIMITY

What we have seen in this chapter is how our culture is permeated by interwoven ideological practices that treat any substantial separation between mothers and infants—and any practices, such as pumping, that are conducive to such separation—as fundamentally compromising motherhood. The fetishization of nursing, and of the special nurturing powers of the proper maternal body, positions mothers as *uniquely* able to meet their children's needs with their proximate, lactating bodies. This helps grant the round-the-clock devotion demanded of mothers the normative sheen of the 'natural.' As we have seen, there is, in fact, nothing natural or even historically typical about positioning mothers as exclusive caregivers and making infants exclusively dependent on their mothers for meeting their basic needs. But, drawing upon the figure of the Fetish Mother, our modern era has constructed a privileged, exclusive relationship between mother and child, cemented by proximity, and has used this relationship as the model and measure of appropriate caregiving. Such practices oppress women in at least two ways.

The first is hard not to notice: an ideology of proximity, which demands such bodily devotion on the part of mothers, dramatically curtails mothers' lived entitlement to engage in activities and projects that are inconsistent with this devotion, and likely often disables mothers with shame, guilt, and inadequacy when they cannot avoid even relatively minor compromises of proximity. (One La Leche League group told a new mother that if she took a weekend vacation without her baby, her baby would think she was dead.)[113] By inducting mothers into a lived and symbolic understanding of mothering as uninterrupted bodily unity and devotion, we clearly make it more difficult for them to carve out a healthy and guilt-free identity of their own, in the midst of the radical upheaval of identity that invariably attends new motherhood. We can expect that ideological practices that use proximity as the fundamental model of motherhood will be especially potent in undermining new mothers' separate identities and projects, as they struggle to make radically new sense of themselves as embodied agents. This is probably often manifested at the psychic level, but in any case it is clearly true at the pragmatic level. A woman who feels that she cannot leave her infant, or even reasonably deny her infant *any* form of access to her body, cannot do the concrete things that normal humans need to do in order to have a meaningful, distinct identity that is comprehensible to themselves and to others.

The second way in which these practices oppress mothers *and* other caregivers is perhaps less obvious. As a culture, we understand and measure the relationship between mother and child in terms of spatial figures of proximity and separation, and we use these figures to understand the boundaries and possibilities of proper mothering. This means not only that we pressure mothers to literally remain next to their infants but also that our whole ability to imagine and evaluate possible mothering and caregiving relationships is shaped by these specific spatial metaphors and figures. An undergraduate philosophy student of one of my colleagues commented in class that she didn't understand how a mother who loved her child could send her to daycare. When she was asked if this meant that fathers, who left the home to work, didn't love their children, she replied that this was a different kind of love. She believed that *only* sustained proximity was consistent with mother-love.[114] This casts mother-love as a *whole different sort* of relationship, with a different shape and different standards, than other kinds of love and caregiving—one in which, unlike in all other human relations, any voluntary separation is a form of betrayal. We assume that healthy, loving relationships between spouses, siblings, or friends include a great deal of separation, and even that each party in such relationships will participate in enabling and enriching their time apart as well as their time together. In fact, in any domain of human relationships other than mothering, the kind of exclusive bodily presence and continuous proximity held as a normative ideal for mothers would be considered deeply problematic and dysfunctional. Yet we rarely question the assumption that proximity is the emblematic measure and means of mothering.

Amy Mullin points out that we tend, as a culture, to measure all caregiving situations by how 'mother-like' they are.[114] Thus, for instance, sending a child to daycare casts suspicion on the mother who is willing to separate from her infant, but also, the daycare situation itself is a suspicious substitute for the mother's care just in virtue of its collective caregiving structure, regardless of whether the children in it are benefiting from the greater stimulation, greater variety and diversity of available caring adults and peers, and more sustained and structured attention compared to what they would receive at home with their mothers. Affluent families often choose a nanny over group daycare, where that nanny's care can more closely simulate the proximate mothering model. Meanwhile, our model of exclusive proximity as the ideal of motherhood casts immediate, often unthematized suspicion upon the mothering practices of ethnic groups that employ more communal forms of child rearing and rely on extended families.[115] I do not have the space here to compare the objective merits (for either children or caregivers) of various forms of caregiving. My contention here is just that we grant higher social cachet to caregiving arrangements that either directly reinforce or simulate sustained, exclusive mother-child proximity, and this cachet is often based on prethematized ideas about what caregiving should look like rather than on informed preferences.

Of course, infants and young children require vastly more direct care and attention, and vastly more physical contact, than older humans, but this does not mean that any *one person* needs to or even should define her relationship to a child in terms of sustained proximity, nor that there should be anyone in the child's life who cannot separate from her without betraying her. Major caregivers—most often mothers—will and ought to have a special kind of intense kinesthetic intimacy with the infants they care for, but this does not mean that this intimacy should be held to a quantitative standard, nor does it mean that it is 'natural' for one person's body to serve as the privileged site of this intimacy, nor certainly that the breastfeeding relationship is the privileged symbol or tool of this intimacy. We have created and fetishized a historically specific and peculiar kind of maternal relationship, governed by quite different normative standards than any other human relationship, and enshrined it as the 'natural' model for appropriate caregiving relationships with infants and young children.

NOTES

1. D. W. Winnicott, "The Baby as a Going Concern," in *The Child and the Family* (London: Tavistock, 1958), 13–17.

2. A. Montagu, *Touching: The Human Significance of the Skin* (New York: Columbia University Press, 1971), 77.

3. Linda Blum, *At the Breast: Ideologies of Breastfeeding and Motherhood in the Contemporary United States* (Boston: Beacon Press, 1999).

4. Mark Eddy Smith, "Nursing the World Back to Health," *New Beginnings* 12(3), 1995, 68–71, 68.

5 American Academy of Pediatrics, "Breastfeeding and the Use of Human Milk: Policy Statement," *Pediatrics* 100(6), 1997, 1035–39, 1035.

6. The press release is available at www.hhs.gov/news/press/2004pres/20040604.html.

7. "101 Reasons to Breastfeed Your Child" at www.promom.org/101/index.html provides an excellent mini-bibliography and summary of the scientific research showing the health benefits of breast milk, although it is a document with its own rhetorical problems.

8. La Leche League International, *The Womanly Art of Breastfeeding*, 6th ed. (New York: Plume Books, 1997), 69.

9. Indeed, the cathection of good mothering onto lactation and nursing is so thorough that adoptive mothers are encouraged to prove their maternal mettle by inducing lactation—an enormously difficult, time-consuming, gadget-intensive procedure with usually modest results at best. The suggestion that this is a valuable use of their time and efforts seems to me to devalue the bodies and maternal commitment and skills of adoptive mothers.

10. The practice of keeping a very young infant against the mother's skin almost constantly, which is a currently in vogue version of proximity as a maternal practice, is known as "kangaroo care"—a title that is interesting for its bestial, prediscursive connotations.

11. Ward, *La Leche League: At the Crossroads of Medicine, Feminism and Religion* (Chapel Hill: University of North Carolina Press, 2000), 86, my emphasis.

12. See Ward 2000, 95 and elsewhere.

13. La Leche League 1997, 12.

14. Cited at Ward 2000, 55.

15. Judith Lauwers and Candace Woessner (Garden City Park, NY: Avery Publishing Group, 1990), 183.

16. Exemplary works in this area include Melanie Klein, "The Importance of Symbol-Formation in the Development of the Ego," in Volume 1 of *The Writings of Melanie Klein*, ed. R. E. Money-Kyrle et al. (London: Hogarth Press, 1975), 219–32; and D. W. Winnicott, *The Child and the Family* (London: Tavistock, 1957).

17. See Janice Doane and Devon Hodges, *From Klein to Kristeva: Psychoanalytic Feminism and the Search for the 'Good-Enough' Mother* (Ann Arbor: University of Michigan Press, 1992), for a good summary of the object relations theorists' construal of the maternal body.

18. Montagu 1971, 81.

19. Chris Bobel, *The Paradox of Natural Mothering* (Philadelphia: Temple University Press, 2002), 62.

20. Blum 1999, 33. Bowlby's program spawned various sympathetic scientific studies in the 1970s (for instance, J. H. Kennel, M. A. Trause, and M. H. Klaus, "Evidence for a Sensitive Period in the Human Mother," *Ciba Foundation Symposium* 33, 1975, 87–101), as well as a scientific backlash attempting to debunk him in the early 1980s (including B. Lozoff, "Birth and 'Bonding' in Non-Industrial Societies," *Developmental Medicine and Child Neurology* 25(5), 1983, 595–600).

21. Naomi Wolf has recently reinscribed this uncritical realism concerning a bond whose all-important existence must be forged on the basis of proximity immediately after birth. See Wolf, *Misconceptions: Truth, Lies and the Unexpected on the Journey to Motherhood* (New York: Doubleday Books, 2001), 37.

22. In an interesting rhetorical twist, Dr. Spock maintains this identification of the natural and the proximate, even while dropping the association between nature and biology. He advises the new mother "to hold her baby in her arms during bottle-feeding, . . . the position that Nature intends." It is the spatial arrangement of the mother and baby that is the mark of normative nature here.

23. For an explicit example of this argument in academic writing, see Sara Quant, "Sociocultural Aspects of the Lactation Process," in *Breastfeeding: Biocultural Perspectives*, ed. P. Stuart-MacAdam and K. A. Dettwyler (New York: De Gruyter, 1995).

24. Bobel 2002, 1, 132.

25. La Leche League 1997, 172.

26. La Leche League 1997, 172.

27. Deutsch, *The Psychology of Women*, Volume 2 (New York: Grune and Stratton, 1945), 294.

28. D. B. Jelliffe and E. F. P. Jelliffe, *Human Milk in the Modern World* (Oxford: Oxford University Press, 1978), 114; cited in Jules Law, "The Politics of Breastfeeding: Assessing Risk, Dividing Labour," *Signs: Journal of Women in Culture and Society* 25(2), 2000, 404–50.

29. D. M. Digman, "Understanding Intimacy as Experienced by Breastfeeding Mothers," *Health Care for Women International* 16(5), 1995, 477–85, 480.

30. Amy Mullin, *Reconceiving Pregnancy and Childcare* (New York: Cambridge University Press, 2005), mss 46.

31. Jules Law argues, "If we see it as a basic feminist premise that the decision whether to continue a pregnancy is a woman's choice and legal right, but that child care is an interpersonal responsibility, . . . then infant feeding clearly lies on the child-care side." Yet, as he suggests, using models and metaphors of pregnancy and mute umbilical cords in order to figure the feeding relationship masks this interpersonal responsibility and insulates practices of infant feeding relationship from critique and articulation (2000, 442).

32. See Valerie Fildes, *Breasts, Bottles and Babies: A History of Infant Feeding* (Edinburgh: Edinburgh University Press, 1986) for a comprehensive history of infant feeding.

33. Pam Carter, *Feminism, Breasts and Breastfeeding* (New York: St. Martin's Press, 1995), 33.

34. Breastfeeding literature also often claims that in some unspecified 'past' or 'primitive' culture, it is/was standard to breastfeed children for much longer than do we Western unnaturals. In fact, Fildes' quantitative data do not bear out this myth. A historical survey shows the normal period of breastfeeding in various past eras of European culture to be anywhere from 6 to 36 months, which roughly accords with our contemporary range (Fildes 1986, 353–54). And African communities, which are disproportionately sentimentalized for their 'natural' breastfeeding practices, show average weaning ages of 15.6 months in cities and 24 months in the country (Fildes 1986, 365), which are later averages than in North America, but again not by any startling amount.

35. Even diapers are sometimes treated as unnatural, ethically suspect intruders between the bodies of mother and infant. Some advocates of "attachment parenting" claim that the real, proper mother, in tune with nature, ought to have developed an acute sensitivity to the infant's body from their prolonged contact so that she can sense when the infant is about to urinate or defecate with enough precision to allow full toilet training by the age of *one month*; anything less proves that the maternal body has fallen short of fetishistic perfection in its unity with the infant. See www.natural-wisdom.com/nihgentlealternative.htm.

36. Nagera, from *Child and Family* 14(2), quoted in La Leche League's "Breastfeeding Rights Packet."

37. Janet Tamaro (Holbrook, MA: Adams Media Corp., 1998).

38. (New York: Bergin and Garvey, 1998), 60, my emphasis.

39. L. Cronenwett, T. Stukel, and M. Kearney, "Single Daily Bottle Use in the Early Weeks Post-Partum and Breastfeeding Outcomes," *Pediatrics* 63, 1992, 760.

40. A. K. Seema-Patwary and L. Satyanarayana, "Relactation: An Effective Intervention to Promote Exclusive Breastfeeding," *Journal of Tropical Pediatrics* 43(4), 1997, 213–16.

41. See in particular C. Fisher and S. Inch, "Nipple Confusion: Who Is Confused?" *Journal of Pediatrics* 129, 1996, 174–75, and the published responses it has generated. Samuel Menahem comments, "Nursery practices have increasingly been altered with an almost evangelical approach by those advocating breast-feeding, at times to the detriment of the baby, mother, or both. This approach, based on questionable data, assumes that if the baby is allowed only to breastfeed, then breastfeeding will be 'more' successful." (Menahem, letter in response to Fisher and Inch, *Journal of Pediatrics* 130(6), 1997, 10–12.)

42. Ruth Lawrence, *Breastfeeding: A Guide for the Medical Profession*, 4th ed. (New York: Mosby Inc., 1994), 268.

43. Tamaro, *So That's What They're For: Breastfeeding Basics* (Avon, MA: Adams Media Corporation, 1998), 126.

44. La Leche League 1997, 73.

45. Eisenberg, Murkoff, and Hathaway, *What to Expect the First Year* (New York: Workman Publishing, 1989), 117–18.

46. See Sara Ruddick's *Maternal Thinking: Towards a Politics of Peace* (Boston: Beacon Press, 1989) for a seminal exploration of the articulated skills of mothering.

47. Blum 1999, 4.

48. This little summary is irresponsibly brief by philosophical standards, but I think it will serve to make my point without harmful distortion in this context. What I have

drawn here is a picture that formed a template for a great deal of seventeenth- and eighteenth-century metaphysics, including that which was shaped by its rejection, such as George Berkeley's idealism. Probably no philosopher was unsubtle enough to be committed to quite the rough picture that I just drew. Descartes would be the most obvious and explicit proponent of such a picture, but even he ought to be read as telling a much more complicated story.

49. I offer the same caveats concerning the dramatic oversimplification that this description represents. Twentieth-century philosophers who did the most to reconceive the nature of human embodiment include Martin Heidegger and Maurice Merleau-Ponty. The philosopher that probably did the most to bring this revision in our understanding of embodiment across the Atlantic was Hubert Dreyfus, especially through his *What Computers Cannot Do* (New York: Harper Collins, 1979) and his *Being-in-the-World: A Commentary on Heidegger's Being and Time Division I* (Cambridge, MA: MIT Press, 1990).

50. For the classic argument against taking mere contiguity as the paradigmatic embodied relationship, see Heidegger's *Being and Time*, Division I, Chapter III (trans. Joan Stambaugh, Albany: SUNY Press, 1996).

51. American Academy of Pediatrics 2002, 159.

52. Tamaro 1998, 28, my emphasis.

53. Law 2000, 424.

54. Weir, "Breasts: Journey from Form to Function," in *The Reality of Breastfeeding* (ed. A. Brown and K. MacPherson, Bergin and Garvey, 1998), 196.

55. Law 2000, 425.

56. Blum 1999, 54–55.

57. The higher IQ of breastfed babies does not seem to depend on how breast milk is delivered; see Lucas A., "Breast Milk and Subsequent Intelligence Quotient in Children Born Preterm," *Lancet* 1992, 39, 261–62. The ephemeral benefits of 'bonding' have been poorly studied and generally do not explicitly look at expressed-milk-fed babies as a group. However, one going theory with some support is that the greater bonding between mothers and breastfed babies is a result of the release of oxytocin during milk ejection, stimulating maternal behavior, and of course pumping produces as much oxytocin as does direct breastfeeding. See Uvnas-Moberg and Eriksson, "Breastfeeding: physiological, endocrine and behavioral adaptations caused by oxytocin and local neurogenic activity in the nipple and mammary gland," *Acta Paediatrica*, 1996, 85(5), 525–30. One of the few studies that does find a correlation between breastfeeding and later psychic well-being (D. M. Fergusson and L. J. Woodward, "Breastfeeding and Later Psychosocial Adjustment," *Paediatric and Perinatal Epidemiology* 12(2), 1999, 144–157) compares breastfed babies only to formula-fed babies, thus leaving it open whether the effect is dependent on proximity, or whether it is perhaps produced by oxytocin or some other factor that is neutral between delivery mechanisms. Furthermore, none of the studies, including this one, control for other forms and amounts of mother-child interaction and contact in comparing breastfed and other babies, even though we would assume that mothers in circumstances that enable breastfeeding may also be in a position that allows them to interact more with their infants in other ways. I have more to say about the problems with the scientific literature on breastfeeding, bonding, and psychic development in the section "The Lactating Body as Scientific Object," below.

58. V. Valdes et al., "Clinical Support Can Make the Difference in Exclusive Breastfeeding Success Among Working Women," *Journal of Tropical Pediatrics* 46(3), 2000, 149–54.

59. New York: Avery Childbirth Reference Series, my emphasis.

60. La Leche League 1997, 62.

61. American Academy of Pediatrics 2002, 203, my emphasis.

62. W. B. Pittard III, D. M. Anderson, E. R. Ceruttu, and B. Boxerbaum, "Bacteriostatic qualities of human milk," *Journal of Pediatrics* 107(2), 1985, 240–43.

63. Most recommendations for sterility practices for bottle feeding draw no distinction between feeding formula and pumped milk, and the precautions that I have just mentioned are actually tailored around formula, which contains none of the antibacterial properties that breast milk has. This elision is itself an example of the silencing and denigration of expressed milk feeding that I am trying to chart.

64. See Pittard et al. 1985; M. T. Asquith, P. W. Pedrotty, D. K. Stevenson, and P. Sunshine, "The Bacterial Content of Breast Milk after the Early Initiation of Expression Using a Standard Technique," *Journal of Pediatric Gastroenterology and Nutrition* 3(1), 1984, 104–10; M. Hamosh, L. A. Ellis, D. R. Pollock, T. R. Henderson, and P. Hamosh, "Breastfeeding and the Working Mother: Effect of Time and Temperature of Short-term Storage on Proteolysis, Liposis, and Bacterial Growth in Milk," *Pediatrics* 97(4), 1996, 492–8; W. B. Pittard III, K. M. Geddes, S. Brown, S. Mintz, and T. C. Hulsey, "Bacterial Contamination of Human Milk: Container Type and Method of Expression," *American Journal of Perinatology* 8(1), 1991, 25–27. Of course, no list of citations can support my claim that *most* of the studies of expressed milk focus on its contamination; an article search is the best way to confirm this.

65. www.promom.org.

66. "Beauty and the Breast," in P. Stuart-McAdam and K. Dettwyler, eds., *Breastfeeding: Biocultural Perspectives* (New York: de Gruyter, 1995), 167.

67. McAdam and Dettwyler 1995, 201.

68. J. Barnes, A. Stein, T. Smith, and J. I. Pollock, "Extreme Attitudes to Body Shape, Social and Psychological Factors and a Reluctance to Breast Feed," *J Royal Soc Medicine* 90(10), 1997, 551–9. For other examples of recent scientific articles that employ the breast/bottle dichotomy, without specifying whether they are controlling for substance or delivery method, and in ways that make the conclusions ambiguous and confusing, see C. L. Wagner and M. T. Wagner, "The Breast or the Bottle? Determinants of Infant Feeding Behaviors," *Clinics in Perinatology* 26(2), 1999, 505–25; R. M. Martin et al., "Association between Breast Feeding and Growth," *Archives of Disease in Childhood, Fetal and Neonatal Edition* 87(3), 2002, 193–201; E. S. Mezzacappa et al., "Breast Feeding and Maternal Health in Online Mothers," *Annals of Behavioral Medicine* 24(2), 2002, 299–309; and E. S. Mezzacappa and E. S. Katlin, "Breast-feeding is Associated With Reduced Perceived Stress and Negative Mood in Mothers," *Health Psychology* 21(2), 2002, 187–93.

69. Smith 1995, 68.

70. www.promom.org.

71. Blum 1999, 46.

72. J. S. Rogers, J. Golding, and P. M. Emmett, "The Effects of Lactation on the Mother," *Early Human Development* 49 sup, 1997, 191–203.

73. Simms, "Milk and Flesh: A Phenomenological Reflection on Infancy and Coexistence," *Journal of Phenomenological Psychology*, 2001, 22–40, 25.

74. See La Leche League 1997; Tamaro 1998; American Academy of Pediatrics 2002; and Murkoff et al.'s *What to Expect in the First Year* for examples of this double message.

75. W. B. Colin and J. A. Scott, "Breastfeeding: Reasons for Starting, Reasons for Stopping, and Problems Along the Way," *Breastfeeding Review* 10(2), 2002, 13–19.

76. We can see the mythic value of breast milk is intimately connected to its *source* and delivery mechanism, rather than its actual chemical composition, in the comment

of one (male!) breastfeeding advocate at a La Leche League conference, who, in response to the purported fact that human breast milk can now be replicated out of mouse milk, claimed that "this advance meant that breastfeeding advocates could no longer promote maternal nursing on the basis of breast milk as a substance. It was time, he argued, to promote breastfeeding as an experience" (Bernice Hausman, *Mother's Milk: Breastfeeding Controversies in American Culture*, New York: Routledge, 2003).

77. Tamaro 1998, 29.

78. Katie Allison Granju, July 1999, at www.salon.com/mwt/feature/1999/07/19/formula/.

79. La Leche League, 1997, 90.

80. www.promom.org, 101 reasons to breastfeed #63.

81. This play on the monstrosity of human-beast hybrids as a complement to the fetishization of breastfeeding again can find roots in Rousseau, who at least maintained consistency by advocating vegetarianism—although, oddly, he insists in *Emile* that women ought to eat lots of dairy products. See my discussion of the significance of hybrids more generally in chapter 3.

82. Dettwyler, in *Breastfeeding: Biocultural Perspectives* 1995, 201.

83. A recent work of art reflects the ongoing depths of our Rousseauian revulsion at the 'unnatural' breast. Two 1994 sculptures by Jean de Buffet, currently installed next to one another in the same case in the Hirshhorn Gallery of Art in Washington, DC, are nearly identical; both are dark, mottled, lumpy masses, looking organic but clearly disorderly. One is called 'Excresance' and the other is called 'Profuse Wet Nurse.'

84. This is admitted and documented in Ruth Lawrence's keystone 1994 textbook *Breastfeeding: A Guide for the Medical Profession*. This text contains a nice summary of the research on breastfeeding up until 1994, as well as the glaring gaps in that research. Yet this same textbook offers a striking manifestation of the apparent immunity of empirical questions about the real relationship between breastfeeding and bonding from the scientific gaze: the textbook includes a chapter entitled "Psychological Impact *of* Breastfeeding," but its content is directly opposed to its title; the chapter is a summary of the impact of psychological factors *on* breastfeeding rates.

85. See for example D. Nitzan Kaluski and A. Levinthal, "The Gift of Breastfeeding: The Practice of Breastfeeding in Israel," *Harefuah* 138(8), 2000, 617–22; and H. E. Lerner, "Effects of the Nursing Mother-Infant Dyad on the Family," *American Journal of Orthopsychiatry* 49(2) 1979, 339–48. There is in fact some evidence that breastfeeding can actually help *delay* very early bonding, perhaps because of the very intensity of new mothers' socially inculcated expectation that breastfeeding will immediately produce bonding and their corresponding disappointment and resentment if this effect is not forthcoming. See J. M. Pascoe and J. French, "The Development of Positive Feelings in Primiparous Mothers towards Their Normal Newborns," *Clinical Pediatrics* 28(10), 1989, 452–56. Pascoe and French do not offer this explanation for their data, but they do find a correlation between reduced attachment behavior and *both* breastfeeding and 'disappointment in the bonding experience.' Furthermore, the focus on primiparous mothers suggests to me a heightened gap between expectations (which for such mothers are not based on firsthand experience) and reality.

86. For an excellent analysis, complementary to mine here, of both the paucity of serious research of the purported emotional and psychic benefits of breastfeeding and the methodologically suspect character of the research that has been done, see Law 2000.

87. R. Tessier et al., "Kangaroo mother care and the bonding hypothesis," *Pediatrics* 102(2), 1998.

88. There is, in fact, evidence that 'kangaroo care'—the practice of keeping the infant against the mother's skin almost continuously—has substantial physical and psychic

health benefits, specifically for very young premature infants. (For example, see R. Feldman, A. Weller, L. Sirota, and A. I. Eidelman, "Testing a Family Intervention Hypothesis: The Contribution of Mother-Infant Skin-to-Skin Contact (Kangaroo Care) to Family Interaction, Proximity, and Touch," *Journal of Family Psychology* 2003, 17(1), 94–107; and A. Conde-Agudelo, J. L. Diaz-Rossell, and J. L. Belizan, "Kangaroo Mother Care to Reduce Morbidity and Mortality in Low Birthweight Infants," *Birth*, 2003, 30(2), 133–34.) But the studies showing this do not draw any distinction in their design between proximity with mothers and with other adults, nor do they separate out breastfeeding as a specific form of proximity per se, so they should not be read as general reaffirmations of the value and significance of the extended nursing maternal body.

89. For a crisp example, see D. A. Fergusson and L. J. Woodward, "Breast Feeding and Later Psychosocial Development," *Paediatric and Perinatal Epidemiology*, 13(2), 1999, 144–57.

90. Dettwyler 1995, my emphasis.

91. This is all apart from the more obvious point that Dettwyler's marshaling support for the importance of breastfeeding from primate studies obscures the fact that civilized human mothers have hugely important and varied ways of physically relating to and nurturing their children that are not available to rhesus monkeys; presumably these forms of relating heavily inflect the emotional and other development of human children and render primate research difficult if not impossible to apply to this particular human domain.

92. American Academy of Pediatrics 2002, 9.

93. American Academy of Pediatrics 2002, 157, 158. Notice that 'Jennifer' does *not* offer her nursling an 'artificial nipple.'

94. I discuss this danger in detail in chapter 6.

95. Indeed, among many contemporary poor women and women of color this association has not died out, and many authors think that this is a partial explanation of lower breastfeeding rates in these populations. For instance, see Blum 1999.

96. Carter 1995.

97. For instance see Carolyn C. Van Blarcom, R. N., *Getting Ready to Be a Mother* (New York: Macmillan, 1932), 164.

98. *Talks to Mothers about Their Babies* (Baltimore: Bureau of Child Hygiene, Maryland State Department of Health, 1923), 14.

99. Van Blarcom 1932, 162, 164.

100. Van Blarcom 1932, 39, my emphasis. The passage continues, "This is, of course, particularly true in the case of those mothers who have not the intelligence, interest, means or time to prepare the artificial feeding in the approved manner."

101. Maryland State Department of Health 1923, 43–44.

102. In La Leche League's guide, they write, "Successful lactation is an expression of a woman's femininity and she doesn't need to count how often she feeds the baby any more than she counts how often she kisses the baby." Peggy Robin perceptively responds, "This sentence contains two troubling implications: 1) the idea that the bottle-feeding mother must be somehow less 'feminine' than a breastfeeding mother, and 2) that . . . quantification is alien to feminine nature" (*Bottlefeeding without Guilt: A Reassuring Guide for Loving Parents*, Rocklin, CA: Prima Publishing, 1995, 126). Here we see a neat implicit opposition between the normative 'feminine' body that does not require quantification and regulation, and the body that for whatever reason falls short of proper feminine virtue—a body that, like the pregnant bodies we saw in the last chapter, must be measured and quantified because of its untrustworthiness.

103. I have not been able to find any qualitative or quantitative systematic research on the kind of early support for breastfeeding that disabled mothers do or do not receive.

It would be very interesting to study the details of the differences (assuming there are some) between how new mothers with disabilities or deformities receive advice and physical support concerning breastfeeding, in comparison with mothers with 'normal' forms and capacities.

104. It is probably also not irrelevant to trends in infant feeding that in the postwar era, when formula feeding became in vogue, women had recently been forced back into domestic space after having been given temporary new freedom and authority in the workplace during the war. It is not surprising that these women would be less comfortable with the unmitigated femininity, domesticity, and lack of mobility that was associated with breastfeeding.

105. For a fascinating and careful study of the cultural and scientific history of infant formula, see Fildes 1986.

106. Carter 1995.

107. La Leche League 1997, 79, 86, my emphasis.

108. Bobel 2002, 15.

109. Ironically, proximity fetishists often 'spiritualize' the physical union of mother and child, contrasting it with the supposedly crass 'materialism' of the culture that would tear the body of the Fetish Mother apart. Women who choose separation from their children in any form are seen as driven by materialist motives, in contrast with the spiritual purity of the choice of proximity. The strange thing is that the reduction of the maternal relationship to a spatial position, and the identification of good mothering with the brute material bond of breastfeeding and perhaps extended skin-to-skin contact, strikes me as a kind of paltry materialism that cannot incorporate (so to speak) the intellectual and emotional and narrative subtlety of good mothering.

110. See Bobel's (2002) discussion of the phenomenon at 88–8s9.

111. I will discuss this type of threat to integrity and identity at great length in chapter 6.

112. Elsewhere I argue that this is in fact the characteristic function of ideology. See for instance my "Talking Back: Monstrosity, Mundanity and Cynicism in Television Talk Shows," in *Rethinking Marxism* 14:1, 2001. My theoretical work on ideology is strongly shaped by Louis Althusser's seminar article "Ideology and Ideological State Apparatuses," in *Lenin and Philosophy* (London: New Left Books, 1971). See also Naomi Scheman's classic feminist article "Anger and the Politics of Naming" (in her *Engenderings*, New York: Routledge 1993) for her excellent philosophical analysis of how emotions can be constituted through social discourse.

113. Robin 1995, 134.

114. My thanks to this colleague for providing the example; I will leave out her name to protect the anonymity of the student.

115. Mullin 2005.

116. See Mullin 2005 for an excellent and sustained discussion of the politics of caregiving.

6

Intimacy, Vulnerability, and the Politics of Discomfort

We human animals each develop a sense of our embodied integrity and boundaries—a sense that is constituted in close relationship with the culture in which we are placed and the risks and possibilities that it offers us—and we grow up with skills, more or less effective, for negotiating these boundaries. These skills and sensibilities help constitute our understanding of who we are and what we can do, along with our actual and felt safety within the concrete social world. A healthy embodied self with sufficient integrity and autonomy is a self that has managed to forge (among other things) a healthy set of bodily boundaries, a space of possibilities for intimacy, a set of distinctions between private and public spaces and activities, and caring involvement with others. The healthy self also inhabits its own body reasonably comfortably, without radical alienation or uncanniness. I propose this list as a list of intuitively necessary (though surely not sufficient) key requirements for what we might think of as the existential health of the embodied self.

New mothers work hard to build or rebuild such a healthy embodied self. Becoming a new mother calls each of these dimensions of embodied health into question and changes its contours. Indeed, new motherhood may seem like an insuperable threat to some of these dimensions of integrity; new mothers may feel that they have lost any claim to private space or to bodily limits, for example, and they may find themselves alienated from spaces in which they were formerly comfortable (such as favorite bars or childless friends' homes) and awkward and insecure in the new spaces in which they must travel (such as pediatricians' offices or 'mommy and baby' playgroups). Phenomenologically speaking, these threats may feel more—or less—dire than they really are. And different women will be differentially successful at building or recovering their integrity, identity, and boundaries after childbirth.

In its social context, the practice of breastfeeding is well positioned to challenge these dimensions of the integrity of the self. The reign of the Fetish Mother demands of us that we give over our bodies, and especially our breasts, to the unfettered consumptive demands of an infant. Our breasts are figured as food, at the same time as they are targets of eroticization and social and physical vulnerability. Public service images portray the edibility of the maternal breast as part of its natural function (see figure 6.1).[1]

Our cultural imaginary asks that our breasts be available to our infants 'on demand'—it insists that we allow infants to consume our bodies, and it denies us the moral standing to feel that we should be able to limit or control this consumptive relationship. But we have been trained for a lifetime before we mother to try to protect our bodies from subjection to the kind of unfettered consumption that breastfeeding, in this context, asks of us. In at least this sense, the terrain of our privacy, and our former, prematernal sense of how to protect and negotiate that terrain and our movement in and out of it, is called into question when we become mothers in general and breastfeeding mothers in particular. Under these circumstances, it would be bizarre if women did not often experience breastfeeding as to some degree a threatening and disempowering practice involving

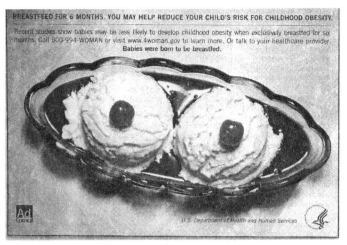

Figure 6.1.   Advertisement from the "Babies were born to be breastfed" campaign, courtesy of The Ad Council, 2004.

vulnerability—a practice that puts them at risk of being exposed, consumed, and violated.

In the previous chapter, I examined how the extended body of the nursing Fetish Mother was governed and sustained by the ideological practices surrounding breastfeeding. There, I scrutinized the ideological practices and representations themselves and how they governed maternal possibilities and behavior. Accordingly, I did not focus on the impact of these practices on the embodied subjectivity of new mothers, from the inside, as it were. However, I believe that living under the shadow of the Fetish Mother has serious implications for new mothers as they renegotiate their experienced and practiced boundaries and integrity, in relation to their infants and in relation to their various communities, intimate and broad, in their new role. The grip of the figure of the Fetish Mother, I will try to show, can be intense enough to leave actual mothers without a realistic or usable model for how to preserve and build their integrity and identity.

The body of the Fetish Mother is seamlessly sutured to the body of the infant. We saw in the last chapter how the Fetish Mother is an important figure guiding our imagination of maternal bodies in all corners of culture, including scientific practice and representations as well as popular imagery. Indeed, the extended maternal body is often treated as a single, unified object of medical attention and management, where the independent character and boundaries of the mother and child are not even given room to appear. In the discourse around early mothering, this unification is often explicit; the 'nursing dyad' and the 'mother-child nursing couple' are often used as singular nouns, while 'maternal-child health' often counts as a single medical specialty.[2] The premier contemporary textbook on breastfeeding contains a chapter called "Managing the Mother-Child Nursing Couple."[3] In trying to understand how to be a healthy self, now that she is a mother in a radically intimate relationship with a being who is overwhelmingly needy and dependent upon her, a woman who looks to this set of cultural resources for help will encounter images of a serene and virtuous maternal body founding order and harmony through her seamless, ecstatic unity with her infant. This does not give her much guidance concerning how to be a loving mother with boundaries and integrity of her own, who can put appropriate limits on her psychic and material availability to her infant, without those limits being damaging or alienating for either her or her infant. In this chapter I will use infant feeding practices as a lens through which to explore some of the challenges that contemporary mothers face when building and sustaining an embodied identity under the shadow of the fetishized maternal body.

WHO WOULDN'T WANT TO BREASTFEED?

Despite widespread outreach and education concerning the substantial and well-established health benefits of breast milk, North American breastfeeding rates continue to be lower than we would hope, especially among low-income women (whose families, we might think, would benefit most from the lower cost and health advantages of breastfeeding) and women of color.[4] While the rates of initiating breast-feeding are now reasonably high among middle- and upper-class white women, even here the rates of continuing to breastfeed for the six months to a year recommended by most medical sources are quite low. In the United States, 65% of new mothers initiate breastfeeding, while only 27% are giving their children any breast milk at all by six months old, and only 12% are doing so at one year old.[5] These numbers raise at least two puzzles from the point of view of breastfeeding advocacy. First, why isn't the information that "breast is best"—a message now disseminated in every form, from this bare slogan through detailed medical information, through health institutions, media campaigns, physicians, nurses, advice books, prenatal classes, websites, outreach programs for mothers at risk, in every language, in Braille, in large font, and in simple words—enough to make mothers choose to breastfeed? How can we avoid the conclusion that the groups of mothers that tend not to breastfeed are just recalcitrantly uneducatable or uncaring? Second, given how we as a culture imagine the experience of breastfeeding—as an ecstatic, joyous, almost spiritual communion between mother and child, providing them with an unparalleled bond—how can we explain the behavior of the millions of women who initiate breastfeeding with every intention of sticking it out for six or twelve months, but quit early? One psychologist ruminates, "it is perhaps surprising, then, that this pleasurable and mutually beneficial experience is disavowed by a large percentage of American women."[6]

Responses to these questions have tended to take two forms. Often, it is simply assumed that despite efforts and appearances, education and information campaigns simply haven't been sufficiently successful in getting their message across, and hence more education and information needs to be disseminated, especially to low-income and minority women. For example, a September 2004 press release concerning the new Health and Human Services breastfeeding advocacy campaign begins, "Not enough U.S. moms are *getting the message* that 'breast is best,'" and backs this up immediately by citing "new statistics" showing that "while U.S. health officials call for mothers to breastfeed their babies exclusively for the first six months of their infants' lives, few mothers actually do so, according to research gathered via CDC's 2003 National Immunization Survey."[7]

Yet studies have shown pretty definitively that women who do not initiate breastfeeding are usually well aware of the benefits of breast milk, and in particular that they are just as aware of them as are their breastfeeding counterparts.[8] Indeed, the original Health and Human Services press release acknowledges, "The United States has one of the lowest rates of breastfeeding in the developed world. . . . Research has shown that many women know that breastfeeding is the best nutrition for their babies. This knowledge has not translated into changed behaviors, and breastfeeding rates have hit a plateau."[9] In the face of this acknowledgment, it is remarkable that the agency's response was to launch another information campaign with a new and hopefully more "compelling" slogan—one which, in their words, will "speak to parents clearly about the consequences of not breastfeeding"[10]—rather than, for instance, question whether abysmal maternity leaves, few workplace protections, and a privatized daycare system may be among the addressable factors explaining the large gap between the infant feeding practices of American women and 'the message' they are given. In the face of the proven distance between U.S. women's infant feeding knowledge and their practices, we need to think carefully about the potential paternalism and imprudence involved in throwing our resources into finding ever simpler, more guilt-inducing, and more repetitive ways of giving women information they have anyhow. We need to question contemporary rhetoric that casts lack of education as itself the *cause* of breastfeeding rather than as a correlate of it that itself needs critical and political analysis and explanation.[11]

A second, more productive set of responses turns to institutional reasons that women have a hard time breastfeeding. Obvious and important examples include insufficient skilled support for overcoming the mechanical difficulties of breastfeeding (such as problems with latch-on, plugged ducts, and so forth), the failure of workplaces and public spaces to make nursing and pumping plausible options for mothers, and the failure of economic systems to make it financially plausible for women to be around their children enough to breastfeed them. Many breastfeeding advocates have worked hard, with substantial but limited success, to get women more of the *material* support they need in order to breastfeed: more accommodation of nursing mothers in the workplace, better access to lactation consultants, better maternity leaves (in countries other than the United States), and so forth. This work is of crucial importance from the point of view of justice and public health, although, as I will discuss later in this chapter, in the details of its implementation it often perpetrates harmful silences and problematic ideology.

What neither of these sets of responses calls into question is the underlying image of breastfeeding as an inherently ecstatic, pleasurable, affirming experience for the mother, as long as she has the physical and economic support she needs. Indeed, it is hard to find much public discourse that would call this assumption into question. Women's subjective experiences of breastfeeding haven't been a topic of much careful empirical attention, and images of the mother's ecstatic pleasure are circulated and reiterated without much concern for their empirical adequacy. In a striking example of this, researchers Janice Riordan and Emily T. Rapp, both also La Leche League leaders, use as an *argument* for the intense pleasurability of breastfeeding the fact that "in perusal of the many paintings of nursing dyads that abound in great collections of art, we may note . . . an expression of pleasure on the mother's face."[12] Here third-person representations of breastfeeding mothers, by male artists who make no pretence to be capturing the concrete rather than the symbolic status of maternal bodies, are treated as transparent evidence of women's subjective states.

Indeed, many women who nurse enjoy perfectly comfortable, pleasurable breastfeeding relationships with their children (although the extremely rapid early drop-off in breastfeeding rates indicates pretty definitively that for whatever reason, many do not). However, if we look carefully we start to uncover a set of concerns and discomforts that form a sharp contrast to the boundary-effacing pleasures of the serene and rapturous Fetish Mother. Some studies have found that sexual abuse survivors have a particularly difficult time breastfeeding. Breastfeeding can trigger abuse memories and post-traumatic stress episodes. Some survivors literally cannot even think about breastfeeding without acute distress. Some may experience irrational rage at normal, playful behavior of their infants during breastfeeding.[13] The secondary psychological impact of these responses on these mothers—for example the potential guilt and shame associated with having these reactions—has not been studied. One study found that women who felt uncomfortable with or disliked their own bodies, or felt anxiety about having sufficient control over their bodies, were less likely to breastfeed.[14] This same study showed that 43% of women who chose not to breastfeed described themselves as finding breastfeeding 'primitive,' 'ugly,' or 'unpleasant' (in contrast to citing more concrete impediments such as physical difficulty or discomfort or difficulties reconciling breastfeeding and working). Low-income women who understand the benefits of breastfeeding often describe it as embarrassing and as a private activity that they cannot accomplish in their crowded homes and workplaces without private spaces.[15]

Therapists who spend a great deal of time enabling women to articulate feelings that may not be socially acceptable or easy to express uncover an even more vivid vocabulary of breastfeeding troubles—a language of discomfort and vulnerability that directly concerns women's experience of their embodied identity and integrity. Some women feel intensely adverse to the experience of having their bodies on call for their infants; they feel their bodies are no longer theirs, and they resent the embodied position of submission in which they find themselves. Some feel that they are engaging in a degrading, incestuous act. Some describe themselves as feeling cow-like and dehumanized by breastfeeding. Some experience anxiety during breastfeeding so intense that they can't bear to hold their children. Some feel crippled by helplessness and fright, both in the face of breastfeeding and in the face of their own reactions to it. It is not uncommon for women to feel raped by their infants during breastfeeding.[16]

As a culture, we have no place or sympathy for the mother who, rather than feeling ecstatic unity during breastfeeding, feels raped, disgusted, angry, or resentful. Hers is not the maternal body from which unity and virtue spring. Scientific literature describes women who do not 'like' breastfeeding as controlling, self-centered, immature, frigid, disengaged, unattached to their infants, and stuck in an oral-sadistic early phase of development.[17] As one article puts it, "The research on personality and breastfeeding suggests that the mother with the ideal *breastfeeding personality* is calm, mature, instinctive, independent, accepting of the giving of oneself, involved in the mothering role, and accepting of the unpredictable nature of childrearing. This woman also is respectful of her own needs and flexible enough to adapt to the frequent demands of breastfeeding. Mothers with contrasting qualities may experience difficulty or discomfort in the breastfeeding relationship."[18] This discourse places the blame for mothers' discomforts firmly on their own individual, psychological, and personality shortcomings and thereby forecloses the space for any more systematic or helpful analysis of these breastfeeding crises and their substantial mental and physical health costs.

We need to ask whether this is the only story to be told about those mothers whose experience is so far removed from the dominant images of breastfeeding. If it is, then mothers who feel deeply troubled by breastfeeding have little hope for revising and healing that relationship, short of radically overhauling their identities and transforming themselves into more 'mature,' 'maternal' beings. But we ought to be suspicious of the pathologization of these women. If there were not already social forces in place that gave special meaning and power to the reasonably physically straightforward act of joining breast to mouth, then it does not seem that even an immature, self-centered, maternally deficient woman would have intense, existentially challenging reactions to this act. A woman's personality alone, however problematic, cannot explain how fraught the feeding of her child can become. Nancy Williams points out that as a culture we "create a powerful mental image of the perfectly beautiful mother sitting in front of the fireplace while violins played and roses created a fragrant room. Seldom do we willingly encourage others to picture their future breastfeeding experience to include traumatized nipples, screaming, back-arching, breast-refusing infants, or hours spent in a love-hate relationship with breast pumps or other gadgets. Reality for most is somewhere between the idyllic and the wrenching."[19] But the distance between images of rapturous maternal ecstasies and the experiences of many women who feel violated, traumatized, or enraged by breastfeeding cannot be explained even by looking to the mechanical difficulties and indignities that breastfeeding can involve, shorn of their imaginative and social significance. In order to understand such experiences, we need to turn critical attention to how the nursing maternal body inhabits a deeply vexed position in the cultural imagination. We already know that the proximity of breast and mouth is a potent normative symbol in our culture, and hence we need to ask how the life of this symbol in the concrete context of contemporary North American society might make breastfeeding traumatic and threatening for some women.

PRIVATE PLACES

Breastfeeding mothers are asked to negotiate an exceptionally complicated and often conflicting set of codes of privacy and publicity. At the very same time as the Fetish Mother is a *public* symbol and locus of virtue and *social* harmony, actual breastfeeding is treated as a *private* activity properly sequestered in an intimate, domestic space. Thus at the same time as nursing is glorified within our social imaginary, real mothers are supposed to obey fairly restrictive codes concerning where, how, when, and in front of whom they breastfeed. The body of the Fetish Mother is a civic, public symbol, and in that sense it is essentially a spectacle. But it functions, in its classic form, as a spectacle of *domesticity* and privacy—of the power of the domestic breast to produce civic virtue and harmonious nature from within the home of the citizen. For an imaginative figure of art and social mythology, the public, spectacular role of this private body poses no contradiction, but it imposes important and complicated restrictions and contradictory meanings upon the real maternal bodies asked to incarnate the fetish ideal.

The breast does not lose[20] its sexualized status in a society that hosts the Fetish Mother.[21] No amount of embodied absorption in new motherhood erases the fact that women's sexuality and sexual vulnerability have important cultural life and meanings. If women breastfeed in public—or, in many women's cases, even in front of their children's father and other caretakers—they risk exposing themselves to sexualized and offended gazes and the dangers that come from each. It has only been in the last twelve years that court rulings in the United States have begun to prohibit charging women who breastfeed in public (no matter how discretely) with indecent exposure—the seminal case was such a ruling in Florida in 1993—and such rulings do not yet have universal jurisdiction, with only a handful of American states currently protecting a woman's right to breastfeed publicly. Indeed, many women, especially poor women and women from ethnic groups that tend to live in more communal and crowded spaces, have literally no safe private space in which they are protected from these gazes. Women from these groups are also more vulnerable in general to sexual abuse and to charges of inappropriate sexual display, and hence they may face intensified risks and more complex codes of privacy when breastfeeding, in comparison with privileged women whose bodies do not challenge dominant norms of femininity and who typically have more mobility and access to privacy.

Although many writers have discussed the double meaning of the breast as sexual object and as source of nourishment, the classic statement on this is R. Rodriguez-Garcia and L. Frazier's 1995 article, "Cultural Paradoxes Relating to Sexuality and Breastfeeding."[22] Here the authors argue that we are widely uncomfortable with this double role for the breast, as 'for' the infant and 'for' sexual pleasure and the (male) sexual gaze. Furthermore, Rodriguez-Garcia and Frazier point out, in taking the maternal and sexual roles of the female body as in tension with one another, we turn the breastfeeding mother's own sexuality into a problem. The vexed double role of the breast not only makes the actual pragmatics of keeping an infant fed awkward, it also transforms the woman's lactating body into the lived site of this incompatibility. One older study showed that men were so uncomfortable with the double role of the breast that in response to questions about their feelings about breastfeeding, they routinely changed the topic to the erotic dimensions of the breast and even told dirty jokes rather than answer the questions.[23] Thus as breastfeeding mothers, women are both sexualized and denied the right to comfortable sexuality. Rodriguez-Garcia and Frazier argue that many women choose not to breastfeed despite knowing its health benefits because they feel that it would be too difficult to keep their nursing sufficiently private and discrete.

Regina Dilgen, who admits in her essay "How I Learned to Stop Worrying and Love the Bottle"[24] that she "remembers breastfeeding as a negative experience"[25] and that in her "memory, the beginning of enjoying motherhood is interwoven with the decision to go with the bottle,"[26] is timid and apologetic about how breastfeeding challenged her sense of privacy and integrity. She writes, "it sounds politically incorrect, but I did not like the intensive care nurses, my husband's grandmother, all of my visitors, seeing my breast. That's mine. Personal."[27] Dilgen describes how she not only craved privacy during breastfeeding but also felt unable to speak up in the face of others' assumptions that this privacy would be unimportant to her; this social bind is echoed in another essay in the same volume as Dilgen's.[28] To the extent that the need for privacy is 'politically incorrect,' mothers are given a radical double message concerning the logic of privacy and boundaries governing our bodies. We are expected to seamlessly incorporate and comfortably accept the double status of our breasts, and of our sexuality more generally, as vulnerable and private insofar as we are women and as a matter of public pride insofar as we are mothers. Yet we have but one body with which to live out and under these conflicting codes.

It would be a mistake to think that the complexity of the codes of privacy and publicity that surround breastfeeding are all directly related to the sexualization of the breast and the female body, although sexuality is probably subtly and inextricably interwoven throughout these codes. The *modesty* demanded of breastfeeding mothers is best understood as the containment of breastfeeding to domestic space, where domestic space is a complex cultural construct that cannot be defined in terms of a literal set of physical spaces. Domestic space is characterized by a set of material arrangements, placements, and boundaries but also by the social life and the kinds of bodies that inhabit it and give it its form, as well as in its segregation from other spaces such as workplaces and public gathering places. Although the majority of North Americans live *somewhere*, and hence have a literal 'domicile,' there are large groups of us that do not have *any* access to the kind of 'proper' domestic space in which breastfeeding is imagined and experienced as nurturing, natural, pleasurable, and appropriate instead of shameful, disgusting, embarrassing, or lewd. Our cultural discomfort with breastfeeding emerges quickly when we leave the imaginary body of the Fetish Mother and her representations and confront real mothers with real lives and breasts trying to feed their children, for whom containment in 'proper' domestic space is difficult, highly oppressive, or even impossible.

Katherine Dettwyler perceptively notes how many of the images of breastfeeding in cultural circulation have a very specific visual rhetoric. She writes, "the images of women breastfeeding their children that are used in infant formula advertising almost invariably show Caucasian women. They are shown breastfeeding newborns or young infants (as opposed to older infants, toddlers or older children), they are pictured wearing modest, frilly, usually white nightgowns or negligees, and the setting is usually a rocking chair in a middle- or upper-class baby's room."[29] We can add to Dettwyler's description that the women in these images are able-bodied, reasonably 'pretty,' and shaped in accordance with social norms for the maternal body—they look neither obese nor undernourished, and their breasts are not unusually large or small.[30] These are women who are marked as 'at home' in canonical domestic space, and this is where we imagine them doing their breastfeeding. I am suspicious of Dettwyler's focus on formula advertisements that use these visual tropes, for I found them to be the hegemonic norm in every kind of text, including breastfeeding advocacy literature and medical pamphlets and guidebooks. In fact, the pervasiveness of this imagery suggests that the entrenched ideology and imagery of the fetishized mother-infant couple cuts robustly across differences in the political and economic interests of those perpetrating breastfeeding images.

Dettwyler argues that formula companies, and our culture more generally, use these images in order to portray breastfeeding as having 'nutritional value only.' This strikes me as a bizarre conclusion, given that intimacy, privacy, proximity, and modest, virginal asexuality seem to be the dominant associations produced by this imagistic tradition. I think that her argument is that these images are designed to make women breastfeed in private and to quit early, doing it only when and for as long as it is nutritionally necessary. But even if the images do causally function in this way, this is not the same as their conveying the message that breastfeeding has only nutritional value. On the contrary, I would argue, these images are integrated into a larger ideology of breastfeeding as involving a specific kind of romanticized unity between mother and child—a union that is protected from the unruly influences of the mundane world, secreted away into a private, domestic, clean, and virginal space. Not only do I read such images as enhancing and supporting the allure of the fetishized nursing maternal couple (whose normative value far exceeds its link with good nutrition), but I think that when formula companies adopt this imagery, they are trying to participate in and metonymically cash in on this allure.

But Dettwyler and I importantly agree that this imagery enforces the containment of breastfeeding to a very specific domain. She points out that "the not so subtle message is that nursing a child is not something one does while dressed in street clothes, not something one does while working, and definitely not something one does with a child old enough to walk and talk."[31] In other words, our modern love affair with breastfeeding is not with the real activity, as an integrated and concrete part of the mobile, multifaceted, and well-rounded lives of mothers, but with a specific fetishized image of breastfeeding, carried out in a private, domesticated domain. As Dettwyler helps us notice, images of the nursing mother usually place her in an *infantilized* space such as a nursery, or a rocking chair invoking a nursery (or else, as in figure 6.2a, the nursing couple is carefully placed in no determinate space at all). The culturally comfortable space for breastfeeding is not one that embodies the contingent complexity and unpredictability of the adult world. It is a controlled, asexual space, designed to be quiet, safe, and free from potentially distressing stimulation. The mother, when placed in this space, is not herself positioned as an independent adult agent but rather as part of the baby's carefully controlled and nurturing environment.

In this sense, La Leche League and the formula companies are in surprising collusion, for both emphasize the importance for breastfeeding mothers of remaining sequestered in such privatized, domestic spaces with their babies. As we saw in chapter 5, La Leche League does advocate 'getting out' with baby, but the space of possible places that they cite as appropriate destinations are all highly gendered and infantilized, including playgrounds, playgroups, and malls. These are, I believe, still domestic spaces in the relevant sense. Just as not all domiciles are properly domestic, likewise not all domestic spaces are domiciles; on the contrary, domestic spaces—gendered, privatized, controlled spaces that are marked as proper sites of maternal nurturance and early child development—can be interwoven through civic space.

Images of mothers in street clothes and busy, public places breastfeeding their children conflict with images that fetishize breastfeeding, by representing the practice as a mundane part of the potentially unruly life of an agent with an autonomous set of activities. It is interesting how even sources that emphasize the possibility of combining work and breastfeeding, and conjure images of moms in smart business suits carrying pumps in discreet 'briefcases,' don't actually include images of mothers breastfeeding at work or even in work clothes.[32] At the same time, the infantilization of the nursing mother (which divests her of her sexuality, drapes her in childlike gowns, and places her in the nursery) helps to mask her adult agency, which is not neatly combinable into a seamless package with the agency of her child.

It is thus not real, multifaceted, unruly mothers with competing projects and independent agency who we trust to breastfeed, but maternal bodies insofar as they are carefully contained and containable within these controlled domestic spaces and can serve as appropriate spectacles of such domesticity. Only such bodies can function imaginatively as incarnations of the Fetish Mother. And we need to keep in mind how the mothers who are most likely not to be in a position to restrict their breastfeeding to the proper, protected, domestic, infantilized domain are low-income mothers and mothers who work at jobs without much enlightened flexibility. Women living in crowded spaces, or at inflexible jobs, or with short maternity leaves, or with houses too small for a dedicated nursery may well be simply unable to fit their nursing bodies into proper domestic spaces, and hence their bodies may be positioned as inappropriate sites of maternity and lactation right from the start.

I have argued that the body of the Fetish Mother is importantly defined in terms of oneness with the infant and that any breach or separation within this body represents a corruption of the maternal bond. We have seen that maternal bodies have long been imagined as having the potential for dangerous unpredictability and untrustworthiness, as well as great power to form human nature through their wombs and their milk. As long as the mother is seamlessly unified with the infant, there is no room for the independent, impertinent, lascivious embodied agency of the unruly mother to play a disorderly formative role. A mother's influence over her child's nature is supposed to be exercised within a controlled space protected from the vagaries and caprice of her body and personality and the chaos of the external world. Her formative power cannot be trusted when she is negotiating the messy everyday world as an independent agent, but only in special circumstances in which her maternal nature can be purified, isolated, and protected from corruption. The domestic domain that I have argued is the proper place of the breastfeeding maternal body is just the kind of space that enables and supports the oneness of mother and infant rather than their potential separation. Formula companies and breastfeeding advocacy organizations such as La Leche League actually share an investment in erasing the possibility of mothers being physically separable from their infants and pursuing their own projects while still providing their children with breast milk, through pumping, supplementing, or otherwise combining work and breastfeeding.

It is rare to find an image of a breastfeeding mother who is looking in any direction other than at her infant; such a look would imply an agency with a direction distinct from the infant's. Although once breastfeeding is established there is certainly no need to stare at the infant throughout the whole process, classic paintings and mothering guides alike stick to images of breastfeeding women whose gaze resolutely maintains the oneness of child and mother. Indeed, even the radical advocacy group that calls itself the 'militant breastfeeding cult,' which supplies a whole set of images for downloading and circulation on its website, sticks closely to this visual trope. In each image except one, a white woman wearing either nothing or a billowy, feminine, virginal gown that is clearly designed for use in private, domestic space, cradles an infant discretely against her body. In each image her breast remains either covered or very abstractly represented, and the infant is held so as to maximize maternal-infant proximity, while the mother keeps her eyes demurely down and gazes at her infant rather than out into the public world, clearly calling up a situation of private intimacy sequestered from the world (see figure 6.2a). The one image they provide that shows a mother looking out at the world as opposed to down at the infant is of an African woman (who is apparently outdoors, unlike the other women pictured) whose body shape and demeanor clearly mark her as a 'tribal,' nostalgic figure irrelevant to contemporary North American practices (see figure 6.2b).

A practice may compromise individuals' agency or autonomy by requiring that they consistently privilege the interests of others over their self-interests. Liberal feminists have long fought against norms of motherhood that demand such compromises and sacrifices from women. But I am arguing here that our cultural understanding of the appropriate breastfeeding body demands an erasure of mothers' independent agency from the start, rather than of her particular interests given that agency. A mother who cannot find an acceptable way to construe herself as separate from her infant at all cannot understand herself as having interests that either coincide or conflict with those of her child. I am not here presupposing any conflicts of interest between mother and child, but instead trying to critique the impact of our cultural imagination of maternal bodies upon mothers' integrity and boundaries.

INTIMACY, VULNERABILITY, AND MATERNAL SEXUALITY

In the last section, I discussed the tension between sexuality and breastfeeding insofar as the maternal body is a sexual or potentially

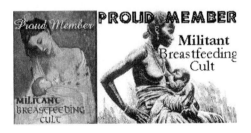

Figure 6.2a, 6.2b. Images courtesy of Militant Breastfeeding Cult, at www.militantbreastfeedingcult .com.

sexual object *for others*. But mothers often experience sexual responses of their own during and through breastfeeding, and these responses are themselves the site of a complicated and vexed set of social meanings and discomforts. Attending to the topic of mothers' own
sexual responses to their infants requires us to peer into a domain that
places the maternal body far outside of the sanitized domain in which
the Fetish Mother resides. It requires that we see the mother not only
as an agent separate from her infant and with her own desires and
boundaries but also as an agent marked by the very feminine sexuality
that has been most traditionally associated with her potential unruliness, and further that we acknowledge that infants and young children
are intimately enmeshed within this unruly sexuality.

Yet it is utterly common for mothers to experience sexual responses of their own during breastfeeding. There are biological reasons
why breastfeeding can trigger sexual arousal in the mother. Suckling
triggers the release of the hormones prolactin and oxytocin, which, in
addition to activating milk ejection, cause uterine contractions. These
contractions and ejaculations are closely linked to the body's responses during orgasm.[33] Indeed, according to self reports—and I think
we should expect a fair amount of underreporting in this area—about
41% of all breastfeeding women experience some form of sexual response during nursing.[34] And even when the physical experience of
breastfeeding has no overtly sexual component, our culture's thorough
sexualization of the breast and the female body, combined with the romantic figures of bodily unity through which we understand breastfeeding, make it likely that mothers will 'read' other kinds of pleasures
and discomforts in breastfeeding as having sexual resonances. This
reading cannot coherently be understood as just an overlay upon an
experience which in its 'pure' form is asexual, for our bodily experiences are always and thoroughly marked and constituted by the socially based understandings we have of those experiences.

Pam Carter writes, "The written texts of breast-feeding are almost
constantly troubled by the demon of sexuality. Various strategic devices to manage this interloper have been adopted. One is to stu-
diously ignore it. A second is to treat the idea that breastfeeding is sexual as a false Western idea. A third is to appropriate breastfeeding as a
heterosexual activity."[35] Katherine Dettwyler marshals the second
strategy, offering the very bad argument that there is no sexual dimension to breastfeeding because the sexuality of the breast is bound
to cultural context and not "intrinsic."[36] Even if we accept her premise, the fact that something is culturally situated and constituted in no
way detracts from its concrete reality.

The first strategy may take the form of simple silence with respect
to sexual dimensions of breastfeeding, but it may also involve the subtler

technique of neutralizing this sexuality through euphemistic transformations of sexual eros into inert pleasure. For example, the American Academy of Pediatrics acknowledges an erotic dimension to breastfeeding only in the form of a single brief reference to the 'fulfillment' and 'physical and emotional communion' that women often experience during nursing.[37] La Leche League sticks to even more veiled and normatively loaded language. They never explicitly mention sexuality, but in a small section entitled "A Pleasurable Experience," we are told that "the mature woman who carries out the totality of her feminine functions knows that she has a niche in the ultimate scheme of things. . . . Breastfeeding is intended to be a pleasurable experience for the mother."[38] The passage insinuates that a mother who does not 'fulfill her feminine functions'—where proper fulfillment requires not only breastfeeding but also experiencing the right kind of pleasure while doing so—has not reached feminine 'maturity' and is not experiencing what she is *supposed to*. Here the erotic dimension of breastfeeding is not suppressed but glorified, but the glorification accesses this eros with the bland language of pleasure, femininity, and maturity rather than the troubling language of overt sexuality.

I think that Carter's first and third strategies are often combined; the erotic dimensions of breastfeeding are inscribed obliquely using heterosexual, highly traditional images of marriage and romantic fulfillment. A *Parents Magazine* article, written in the first person, reports that "nursing is a sort of marriage, an intimate bond between two separate beings, and I wanted a private honeymoon."[39] In one online article, another mother writes, "Joey latched on and happily nursed until he drifted off to sleep. . . . Adrenaline pumped through my system, as excitement, joy and satisfaction swept over me. I was soaring. My baby was still my baby. He still wanted me. We were whole again."[40] Another first-person account, this time in *Mothering* magazine, reports somewhat more explicitly, "I'm in love with the little guy, head over heels, what can I do. He can get my bra off faster than anyone I ever met, no hands at all, just a hungry look."[41] And with remarkable directness, a scholarly article entitled "Completing the Female Sexual Cycle" asserts, "Beginning the mother-baby relationship without lactation is like beginning the marriage without coitus."[42]

Such representations figure breastfeeding as involving a harmonious erotic *union* of mother and infant that is smoothly modeled using the normatively palatable language of heterosexual romance between adults—a kind of sanitized 'love affair,' which eliminates or overcomes the boundaries between the two bodies through joyous, ecstatic pleasure. In every quotation I found that used the metaphors and language of romantic love in order to describe the eros of breastfeeding, the infant was always explicitly marked as male. To see how our implicit heteronormative model of appropriate sexual response is mobilized in our response to these references to maternal-infant eros, notice how odd and jarring this last quotation (about removing the mother's bra with a hungry look) would be if it marked the infant as female instead of male.

I have argued that when nursing mothers display their separate identities and boundaries from their infants, their bodies become unacceptable and problematic. Sexuality within the breastfeeding relationship is acceptable insofar as it is or can be neatly construed as a reaffirmation of the romantic 'oneness' of mother and child. For example, our promotion of a bland, romanticized image of the pleasures of breastfeeding young infants exists alongside our deep cultural disgust at the breastfeeding of older children. We are especially uncomfortable with children's own verbal expressions of their desire to breastfeed. It is odd that we insist that breastfeeding is an essentially pleasurable and affirming event for mothers and young infants, while a child who can articulate a personal desire for this pleasure strikes us as problematic. I suggest that this is because this articulation makes manifest the desire *of* one agent *for* satisfaction from the body of another. At this point, the union of the mother and child by way of the breast can no longer be glossed as a simple, mute unity of two bodies. Similarly, to the extent that a mother's sexually charged response to her child reveals itself in a way that discloses her as separate from this child, marked by independent desires and vulnerabilities, this sexuality becomes highly unacceptable and threatening. The mundane, unruly mother with her own agency and sexuality, who lets her infant suckle at her breast, risks deforming her child into a monster or a pervert.

Denise Perrigo was a La Leche League member and single mother who was a strong believer in the importance of breastfeeding her children. One day in January 1991 she put in a frantic call to a community service center that connected people in crisis with appropriate hotlines. She was distressed because she had experienced some sexual arousal while breastfeeding her toddler, and this arousal felt inappropriate and scary to her. She asked to speak to a La Leche League consultant so that she could talk about whether these feelings were normal and whether she should do anything about them. (It is significant that she did not already know that these feelings were normal, even though she had been regularly attending La Leche League meetings for years.) But the call center volunteer, hearing Perrigo mention being aroused by contact with a child, transferred her without her knowledge to a rape crisis hotline instead. The person who talked to her there called the police immediately and her home was raided. Her toddler was forcibly removed from her care, and she was put on trial as an unfit mother. During the trial she was portrayed as a sex addict in need of discipline and rehabilitation for her lack of sexual control. It took her a year to regain custody of her child, and after this her mothering and lifestyle remained under intense, long-term state scrutiny.[43]

This case has several interesting features for my purposes. First, it is clear that Perrigo broke crucial social taboos with respect to which discomforts we are allowed to voice, with punitive repercussions. Second, we see in the Perrigo case how the body of the Unruly Mother lies in the shadow of the body of the Fetish Mother. Perrigo was put on trial for being *overly* sexual, for not being able to control her sexuality, even though she had called for advice specifically because she was disturbed by her very normal sexual responses and hence was if anything displaying sexual timidity. When the normal sexual arousal of nursing is contained within the rhetoric of organic, romantic oneness with the infant, it is not treated as indicative of excessive or unruly sexuality of the sort needing surveillance and discipline. But when this same arousal is voiced in a way that marks the separation of the mother from the infant—when, as in Perrigo's case, it raises questions about maternal boundaries, privacy, and desires—then it is received as threatening and monstrous. As a breach in the sealed, fetishized maternal body emerges, the mother crosses over to the side of the unruly, and her body becomes a threat to the child's nature, a force that may disfigure and pervert the child rather than nurture it. Perrigo's case gives the lie to any idea that the sexual dimension of breastfeeding is immune from the dangers and vulnerabilities that constitute the terrain of female sexuality more generally.

Romantic descriptions of maternal-infant sexuality and intimacy as inherently organic, natural, pleasurable, and affirming mask the possibility that any threat, discomfort, or boundary violation could be involved in the erotic encounter between mother and infant. But sexuality is a multidimensional, enculturated phenomenon, rife with tensions and conflicts and power differentials. This is as essential to the erotic terrain of human life as is the possibility of romantic union and ecstasies. Furthermore, even as it is marked as appropriately private, it is a relationship that is subject to public scrutiny, judgment and control. In sharp contrast to the mother on the 'private honeymoon' or the mother who was in love with her hungry, bra-removing son, one mother admits in an anonymous interview, "I'm just not comfortable with the idea of breastfeeding. This may sound silly, but I just can't help thinking of my breasts as being sexual. The idea of a baby manipulating them seems almost . . . incestuous."[44] And another mother says "sometimes . . . I really feel physically violated, especially when my son paws at me; I mean, I just can't express it any other way . . . then of course, at the end of the day when my husband gets a little romantic, I just feel like 'don't touch me.'"[45] Remember that in therapy, also, women describe themselves as being raped by their infants, and that discomfort with breastfeeding is associated with survival of sexual abuse.

We often leave unchallenged the assumption that breastfeeding is an inherently pleasurable experience, and that if only the rest of the world would be more supportive of breastfeeding per se, all (normal, maternal) mothers would be free to experience the ecstatic union enshrined in the figure of the Fetish Mother. But in fact, there is no such thing as the *pure* character of the breastfeeding experience, which can be extracted and isolated from the overlay of experiences due to social responses and attitudes. The lived phenomenology of breastfeeding does not divide into those components that issue from the mother's 'personal' relationship to the practice and those that issue from her response to social attitudes and pressures. Rather, positioned as it is as a practice within cultural meanings and institutions—which is the only kind of practice that exists and has any determinate character at all—mothers' own personal experience of breastfeeding and of their relationship to their infant during breastfeeding will be ineliminably marked (though of course not completely determined) by the social position of this practice.

Cristina Traina astutely points out that "some women experience considerable conflict, even revulsion, at experiences of arousal during breastfeeding, or even at sharing their breasts—which had for them been organs of sexual pleasure or display—with an infant. . . . How 'natural' following 'nature' is depends on whether our experience permits us to trust it."[46] In the context of a society in which sexual interactions for women come along with all sorts of risks, there is no reason to think that it would be rational or likely that women would always enter into these interactions trustfully. We need to remember that taking a liberated attitude toward erotic pleasure cannot erase the fact that sexuality and eros live within the interstices of a culture of power, inequality, and vulnerability, and not all women are in a position to take their own sexual responses as safe or pleasurable. And those sexual responses that are fraught with risk or marked as abject can be experienced as violating, scary, or disgusting.

Resources for breastfeeding women and representations of breastfeeding often undermine the articulation of any such discomforts simply through their committed silence on the topic. La Leche League's guide has an entry in its index for 'Breastfeeding—Pleasurable,' but no corresponding negative entry. The guide mentions the possibility of actual unhappiness with breastfeeding—as opposed to physical roadblocks to an eventual pleasurable breastfeeding relationship for the perseverant mother—in only one sentence, in the brief section on postpartum depression. Here, unhappiness with nursing is treated as symptomatic of maternal pathology. Indeed, both the La Leche League and the American Academy of Pediatrics guides, along with various less authoritative lay sources, claim that breastfeeding generally serves to ward off or even cure postpartum depression. In fact, however, systematic studies have not found any strong or consistent correlation of any sort between breastfeeding practices and maternal depression, with some studies showing no correlation, some showing marginally more depression among breastfeeding mothers, and some marginally less.[47]

The Womanly Art of Breastfeeding introduces breastfeeding with a second-person, present-tense description of 'your' idyllic first encounter with your infant, to which your relaxing, pleasurable, meaningful first breastfeeding experience is integral.[48] The grammar of the passage leaves no room for a different experience of this first encounter:

> The umbilical cord is cut, marking the first separation. Who is to bridge this change of worlds for your newborn, who will soothe him and let him know he is again secure? Who better than his mother? Again your body cradles him. You touch him, kiss his cheek, stroke his damp little head. Will he nurse? Perhaps. At some time during the first hour or so he will take the breast. You hold him close and he nuzzles your breast. His tiny mouth grasps your nipple. It seems no less than amazing! You and your baby can relax. After the enormous effort of giving birth, this is sweet reward.

The only emotional experiences mentioned in the 250-page American Academy of Pediatrics breastfeeding guide are "joy," "fulfillment," and "emotional communion." Interestingly, this guide acknowledges the potentially problematic connection between breastfeeding, privacy, and sexuality only as a problem for *fathers*. In the chapter called "The Father's Role," the guide 'quotes' a father who says, "all of a sudden, my wife didn't want to be touched anymore—ever. That was the hard part of adjusting to parenthood, but now we're back the way we were."[49] This passage takes what sounds like a serious crisis of boundaries and embodied comfort for the mother and transforms it into a minor and quickly resolved challenge *for the man* who is used to having sexual access to her.

Lactation consultants and other health providers are primarily trained to look for mechanical explanations of nursing problems, and hence they will understandably be inclined to interpret mothers' discomforts and worries in these terms and to assume that a mother who is not experiencing any mechanical roadblocks has 'no reason' to have a problem with breastfeeding. Often, then, when women's discomforts with breastfeeding do emerge, they are quickly countered with advice that closes off issues of sexuality, integrity, vulnerability, and anxiety in favor of more familiar issues such as latch-on and plugged ducts. This sidestepping is actually recommended by the textbook *Counseling the Nursing Mother*, whose authors write, "many women . . . are vaguely uncomfortable with the whole process [of breastfeeding]. . . . You can help these women by giving them information about the advantages and disadvantages and the techniques used while breastfeeding."[50] This passage places absolutely no value on trying to listen to, clarify, or address these vague discomforts. Indeed, despite the fact that this is a counseling textbook, this is its only mention of how to address mothers' own attitudes toward or feelings about breastfeeding. In this text, the section on breastfeeding problems is divided into two subsections, entitled "concerns related to the baby" and "concerns related to the breast." This division does not allow room in the text for concerns related to the mother as a whole person (and not just one of her body parts), and hence it forecloses issues concerning how she, as a person, is negotiating the breastfeeding relationship.

In a 1963 breastfeeding guide, Karen Pryor planted the blame for discomforts during breastfeeding squarely upon the deficient individual personality of the mother: "An occasional truly neurotic mother, breastfeeding against her real wishes, cannot give herself to her baby at all. There are, after all, frigid breastfeeders, just as there are frigid wives."[51] Pryor's unforgiving language is actually quite helpful, for it leads us to notice an important analogy. Talk of 'frigid wives' has become unacceptable. We now recognize that women who 'cannot give themselves' to their husbands are not necessarily 'truly neurotic' but may be positioned in such a way that this giving is not a gift but a violation of their safety and boundaries. A wife who is not willing to provide her husband with access to her body on demand is not necessarily inherently unloving or dysfunctional. And, we understand now, there is a myriad of politically important reasons why a specific wife may be unable to find pleasure or trust in her sexual relationships. But we have not thought through the need to extend this political understanding to women who find breastfeeding disturbing and challenging rather than pleasurable.

Denise M. Digman, in "Understanding Intimacy as Experienced by Breastfeeding Mothers," identifies intimacy uncritically with union, harmony, reciprocity, joy, closeness, connectedness, and trust.[52] But intimate contacts are often the sites of risk and boundary violations, most obviously but not exclusively for women. If we understand intimacy only as a kind of *union* of selves, we leave no room for how intimacy can involve close contact between two selves with distinct boundaries and hence carry a special risk of violating these boundaries. Without boundaries, no violation is possible, but with boundaries, intimate contact is just where violation is most possible. Pam Carter perceptively points out that the "lack of apparent concern with breast-feeding [among most feminists] is in marked contrast with extensive feminist attention to other areas of women's health and reproduction. . . . With very few exceptions, feminist energy in relation to the politics of breastfeeding has provided little challenge to the mainstream preoccupation: how to get more women to breastfeed longer. The problem of declining breast-feeding rates has almost universally been seen as an assault by baby-milk manufacturers on women's natural capacities."[53] In other domains, feminists have made it clear how intimate relationships, prominently including sexualized relationships, are far from protected from the power dynamics that inflect the public sphere. And they have brought home the ways in which the trust and vulnerability that are put so vividly into play in sexual encounters are themselves socially situated and often dangerous for women. Thus it is surprising that the intimacy involved in breastfeeding has not come under much feminist scrutiny or critique. So far, feminist discourse has not really helped women to understand that their hard-won right to protect their sexualized bodies and boundaries is a right that they should still be able to claim as mothers.

Many scholars and activists concerned with the social position of the maternal body emphasize the importance of creating safe spaces for mothers' expression of their sensual enjoyment of breastfeeding.[54] I take no issue with this as a political goal in and of itself; however, it seems to me that it is at least as important, for political and for public health reasons, that we create safe spaces for mothers to express their discomforts and displeasures with breastfeeding. We have created a culture in which women's bodies and boundaries are vulnerable and their experience of sexuality is fraught with ambivalence, and we have placed upon the breasts of these bodies a mythically proportioned responsibility for the physical and moral well-being of children and societies. But at the same time we offer no tolerance, support, protection, or public voice for women who experience vulnerability or ambivalence while nursing and mothering. An environment that silences or pathologizes the possibility of genuine breastfeeding discomforts and insists that breastfeeding will be an ecstatic pleasure once mechanical hurdles are crossed, is likely to reinforce such mothers' experience of themselves as abject, inappropriate, unmotherly, and incapable of negotiating their embodied relationship to their infants in healthy and sustaining ways.

MAKING SPACE

Safe places in which we can negotiate our *separateness* from our children are at least as necessary as safe spaces in which we can celebrate and give voice to the joys of oneness with these children. Denise Perrigo's case exemplifies in extreme form an occasion where such safety was missing. But making the right kind of safe space for mothers seems to require a major overhaul of deeply entrenched ideologies and practices surrounding the management of maternal bodies. This is not a plausible or concrete short-term goal, so we need to think on a smaller scale about appropriate and inappropriate means for responding to maternal discomforts, *given* that these discomforts are situated in culture that both helps constitute them in the first place and also refuses to acknowledge or support them

The emphasis in health and community organizations on repackaging and redistributing the message that "breast is best" seems misguided. The repetition of this message to a woman who is struggling with breastfeeding reinforces her shame at not having a successful breastfeeding relationship without providing her with any tools for building one. More generally, we need to correct the overwhelming extent to which our methods for responding to breastfeeding difficulties focus on trying to 'fix' the mother herself, either by giving her information or by trying to correct her personality, rather than on identifying, understanding, and changing the socially embedded status of breastfeeding. Health providers need to patiently participate in the project of articulating the discomforts and challenges to healthy embodied selfhood that women may struggle with when they become nursing mothers.

Margaret Little has argued at length that commitments whose fulfillment essentially involves the negotiation and penetration of the intimate boundaries of the embodied self require a different moral discourse and conceptual framework than do duties that can be construed as contract-like obligations between well-bounded, fully separate individuals.[55] Previous discussions of the ethics of breastfeeding have usually been cast either in terms of the competing rights of mother and child—the right to mobility and self-determination vs. the right to health and nurturing—or in terms that deny that breastfeeding might pose a morally significant problem for anyone concerned. I hope to have shown that breastfeeding is a more complex moral terrain than either of these options allows. A simple affirmation of the mother's rights over her own body does not in any way illuminate the morally complicated negotiations of boundaries and integrity and care and nurturance that early mothering can involve; such an affirmation takes this body and its boundaries as a given and then worries about its moral status, rather than seeing the moral complexity in mapping out the boundaries of the body in the first place—especially a body as volatile and under negotiation as the body of a new mother. A simple affirmation of a mother's duty to breastfeed, meanwhile, treats breastfeeding as an act by a moral agent whose status and obligations are fixed in advance—an act perhaps compelled by, but ultimately external to, the identity of the mother as a moral agent—rather than recognizes how the moral contours of the mother's agency and identity are themselves at stake and under negotiation.

I do not, in fact, believe that mothers have an obligation to breastfeed—neither an absolute duty, nor even an obligation that can be entered into something like a summative calculus of obligations. But I do think that mothers, health care providers, and others have a moral and social responsibility to work to orient ourselves in such a way that breastfeeding becomes less threatening and more sustainable. For mothers, this means making a decent effort to find a way to sustain breastfeeding while maintaining their integrity and building pliant but sustainable boundaries. For us as a culture, this means creating public spaces that support breastfeeding, particularly in its mundane, imperfect, sometimes unpleasant, nonfetishized forms, in recognition of mothers' need for independent agency and for substantial boundaries that separate them from their children. For health care providers, this means taking responsibility for hearing and helping to interpret the discomforts of early motherhood, without trivializing them, pathologizing them, deferring responsibility for responding to them, or translating them into mechanical difficulties.

In general, we need to adopt a critical rather than an unreflective participatory stance toward the myths, figures, and ideologies that govern our imagination of maternal bodies. We need to *demystify* the maternal body and the milk it produces and to undermine the mythologies of the maternal body's magical powers, both good and evil. Furthermore, we need to educate women (both practically and theoretically) about the (realistic) health benefits of breast milk, the various ways of getting milk to their children, the difficulties they may face in doing so, and the irrelevance of these difficulties to their suitedness to mothering. This would be an important step toward enabling more women to find a form of embodied interaction with their children that allows both to flourish as independent but deeply bonded beings. In a context where maternal bodies are not so vulnerable or so quick to be deemed unruly, dangerous, or unmotherly; where women's sexual privacy and boundaries aren't continually threatened; where mothers aren't penalized for struggling to define personal boundaries— in such a context, breastfeeding would certainly be a less vexed, more sustainable, healthier option in the first place for many women.

NOTES

1. This image, which is part of the new "Babies were born to be breastfed" campaign (see chapter 5), is especially remarkable for the visual contradictions it offers. It represents the 'natural' breast through an image of maximally unnatural food, with maraschino cherries for nipples, and it represents the purported ability of the maternal breast to nourish without causing obesity with a fat-and-sugar-filled, nearly nutrition-free ice cream sundae.

2. See Peggy Robin, *Bottlefeeding without Guilt: A Reassuring Guide for Loving Parents* (Rocklin, CA: Prima Publishing, 1996), 133.

3. Ruth Lawrence, *Breastfeeding: A Guide for the Medical Profession*, 4th ed. (New York: Mosby Inc., 1994).

4. For a comprehensive list of citations on this topic, see Nurit Guttman and Deena R. Zimmerman, "Low-Income Mothers' Views on Breastfeeding," *Social Science and Medicine* 50, 2000, 1457–73, and for an excellent critical discussion of the reasons why women from these groups breastfeed less, see Linda Blum, *At the Breast* (Boston: Beacon Press, 1999), chapter 5.

5. According to the most recent figures from the American Academy of Pediatrics and the Center for Disease Control and Prevention, National Center for Health Statistics. Also see the Ross Mothers Survey at www.ross.com/aboutRoss/Survey.pdf for information on breastfeeding rates.

6. Harriet E. Lerner, "Effects of the Nursing Mother-Infant Dyad on the Family," *American Journal of Orthopsychiatry* 49(2) 1979, 339–48.

7. *The Nation's Health* 34(7), September 2004, 4.

8. See for example Guttman and Zimmerman 2000.

9. www.hhs.gov/news/press/2004pres/20040604.html.

10. www.hhs.gov/news/press/2004pres/20040604.html.

11. A clear recent example is M. Ummarino et al., "Short Duration of Breastfeeding and Early Introduction of Breastmilk as a Result of Mothers' Low Level of Education," *Acta Paediactrica*, 92, 2003, 12–17. Despite its title, the study upon which this article reports does not make any effort to show such a causal rather than correlative relationship between low education and what the authors call 'infant feeding malpractice.' Furthermore, the article reports on the fact that the low-education mothers received the same information from their pediatricians about the benefits of breastfeeding and the

same instructions about the introduction of cows' milk as their better-educated peers, but it does not take this fact as itself requiring an explanation that might problematize their suggested *causal* relationship between ignorance and 'feeding malpractice'; instead, it merely calls for greater awareness among pediatricians that low-income women may be "noncompliant" when it comes to feeding instructions.

12. Riordan and Rapp, "Pleasure and Purpose: The Sensuousness of Breastfeeding," *Journal of Obstetric and Gynecological Neonatal Nursing* 9(2), 1980, 109–12.

13. See Kathleen Kendall-Tackett, "Breastfeeding and the Sexual Abuse Survivor," *Journal of Human Lactation* 14(2), 1998, 125–30; and J. A. Roussillon, "Adult Survivors of Sexual Abuse: Suggestions for Perinatal Caregivers," *Clinical Excellence for Nurse Practitioners* 2(6), 1998, 329–37.

14. S. F. Foster, P. Slade, and K. Wilson, "Body Image, Maternal Fetal Attachment and Breast-Feeding," *Journal of Psychosomatic Research* 41(2), 1996, 181–84.

15. Guttman and Zimmerman 2000.

16. From conversations with licensed therapists Stephanie Irwin, Laurence Kirmeyer, and Leslie Smith, 2001, 2003.

17. See Lerner 1979; Foster et al. 1996; J. Barnes et al., "Extreme Attitudes to Body Shape, Social and Psychological Factors, and a Reluctance to Breast Feed," *Journal of the Royal Society of Medicine* 90(10), 1997, 551–59; and M. H. Kearney, "Identifying Psychosocial Obstacles to Breastfeeding Success," *Journal of Obstetrical, Gynecological and Neonatal Nursing* 17(2), 1988, 98–105.

18. Kearney 1988.

19. Nancy Williams, "Maternal Psychological Issues in the Experience of Breastfeeding," *Journal of Human Lactation* 13(1), 1997, 57–60, 57.

20. There is a small literature that debates whether this sexualization of the breast is part of human nature or a social construction—see for example Riordan and Rapp 1980 and K. Dettwyler, "Beauty and the Breast," in *Breastfeeding: Biocultural Perspectives*, ed. P. Stuart-MacAdam and K. A. Dettwyler (New York: De Gruyter, 1995). In contrast with, for instance, Dettwyler, I can't actually imagine how this debate matters to the ethics of breastfeeding practices. If the sexualization of the breast is socially constructed, it's not a social construction that is likely to be deconstructed anywhere near here in time or place.

21. Indeed, Joan Landes shows how the eroticization of the breast was a vehicle of the political force of many of the images of the bare-breasted or nursing Republic. See Landes, *Visualizing the Nation: Gender, Representation and Revolution in Eighteenth Century France* (Ithaca: Cornell University Press, 2001).

22. *Journal of Human Lactation* 11(2), 111–115.

23. Cited in Lerner 1979, 342. I assume that consciousness has been sufficiently raised since the 1970s that many fewer men would directly respond in this way. However, it is clear that the double role of the breast is still problematic for the male gaze. In a 2002 episode of the hugely popular and trendy sitcom "Friends," one of the male characters watches his female friend, to whom he is very sexually attracted, nurse her newborn. The physical comedy that carries the scene is based on portraying this as a form of torture for the male friend, who can't bear to look at his friend nursing, even though she is not uncomfortable with the display.

24. Brown, A. and K. MacPherson, eds, *The Reality of Breastfeeding* (New York: Bergin and Garvey, 1998). As I mention in the section Private Places, Dilgen's is one of two essays out of over fifty in this book that describe breastfeeding as a negative experience overall.

25. Brown and MacPherson 1998, 46.

26. Brown and MacPherson 1998, 58.

27. Brown and MacPherson 1998, 47.

28. By Keren Giles, the one other author who gives a negative account of breast-feeding.

29. Dettwyler 1995, 190.

30. An interesting example is the American Academy of Pediatrics guide to breast-feeding, AAP, *New Mother's Guide to Breadfeeding* (New York: Bantam, 2002), which includes many drawings of nursing mothers, all of whom are marked as either Caucasian or racially ambiguous, and all of whom have canonically acceptable body shapes and features. This same guide contains only a handful of drawings of fathers, and two of them are clearly not Caucasian, while one is obese.

31. Dettwyler 1995, 190.

32. Gabrielle Palmer's book *The Politics of Breastfeeding* (London: Pandora Press, 1988) is the classic examination of the socio-symbolic incompatibility of breastfeeding and work.

33. M. D. Avery, L. Duckett, and C. R. Frantzich, "The Experience of Sexuality During Breastfeeding among Primiparous Women," *Journal of Midwifery and Women's Health* 45(3), 2000, 227–37.

34. Avery et al. 2000, 232.

35. Pam Carter, *Feminism, Breasts and Breastfeeding* (London: MacMillan, 1995), 135.

36. Dettwyler 1995.

37. American Academy of Pediatrics 2002, 10.

38. La Leche League, *The Womanly Art of Breastfeeding*, 6th ed. (New York: Plume Books, 1997), 377.

39. Quoted at Blum 1999, 4.

40. Quoted at Robin 1996, 136.

41. *Mothering*, Spring 1995, 88. Although this passage is supposed to reflect delight, a careful reader might be disturbed by the images of passivity, subjection, and consumption used here to articulate erotic union.

42. A. Coleman and L. Coleman. "Completing the Female Sexual Cycle: Intercourse, Childbirth and Breastfeeding," *Sexual Medicine Today*, 2(5), 1978, 34–40.

43. The facts of the Perrigo care are easily available from multiple sources.

44. From an interview in Robin 1996, 67.

45. Blum 1999, 99.

46. C. Traina, "Passionate Mothering: Toward an Ethic of Appropriate Mother-Child Intimacy," *Annula of the Society of Christian Ethics*, 1998, 82.

47. For an example of each result, see J. M. Pascoe and J. French, "Development of Positive Feelings in Primiparous Mothers toward Their Normal Newborns: A Descriptive Study," *Clinical Pediatrics*, 28(10), 1989, 452–56; T. O'Neill, P. Murphy, and V. T. Green, "Postnatal Depression—Aetiological Factors," *Irish Medical Journal* 83(1), 1990, 17–18; and T. A. Papinczak and C. T. Turner, "An Analysis of Personal and Social Factors Influencing Initiation and Duration of Breastfeeding," *Breastfeeding Review* 8(1), 2000, 25–33. Significantly, new mothers' depression is apparently much more dependent upon their *expectations* about feeding, and their feelings of success or failure in the feeding relationship, than upon what or how they feed their infants. See K. E. Pridham et al., "The Relation of a Mother's Working Model of Feeding to Her Feeding Behaviour," *Journal of Advanced Nursing* 35(5), 2001, 741–50.

48. La Leche League 1997, 5. This passage brings together a plethora of the rhetorical strategies and tropes I have been exploring in the last few chapters—the manipulative and normalizing use of the second person, the use of the figure of the umbilical cord as a metonymic introduction to the breast-mouth relation, the emphasis on quickly clos-

ing and suturing separation, the unique power and responsibility assigned to the maternal body, and, most relevant right here, the foreclosure of the possibility that breastfeeding will not be smooth and pleasurable.

49. American Academy of Pediatrics 2002, 219.

50. Judith Lauwers and Candace Woessner, *Counseling the Nursing Mother: A Reference Handbook for Health Care Providers and Lay Counselors* (Garden City Park, NY: Avery Publishing Group, 1990), 181.

51. Quoted in Julie DeJager Ward, *La Leche League: At the Crossroads of Medicine, Feminism and Religion* (Chapel Hill: University of North Carolina Press, 2000), 40.

52. In *Health Care for Women International*, 16(5), 1995, 477–85.

53. Carter 1995, 1.

54. See Miriam Yalom, *A History of the Breast* (New York: Ballantine Books, 1997), and Blum 1999 for two prominent examples.

55. Little, *Compelling Intimacy: Abortion, Law, and Morality*, forthcoming from Oxford University Press.

7

Fixing the Boundaries
of Mothers' Bodies

THE DARK BUT FIRM WEB OF EXPERIENCE

> In the last years of the eighteenth century, European culture outlined
> a structure that has not yet unraveled; we are only just beginning to
> untangle a few of the threads, which are still so unknown to us that
> we immediately assume them to be either marvelously new or ab-
> solutely archaic, whereas for two hundred years (not less, yet not
> much more) they have constituted the dark, but firm web of our ex-
> perience.[1]

So closes Foucault's *The Birth of the Clinic*. In this book I have tried
to show how the medical, social, and phenomenological structure of
the maternal body is likewise neither "marvelously new nor absolutely archaic" but instead grounded in the intellectual, political,
and scientific revolutions of the eighteenth century. Many contemporary scholars studying feminine and maternal bodies, despite their explicit distaste for 'binary oppositions,' tend to presume that we have
only two options: we can treat the character of the body as 'natural' or
'objective' in the sense of ahistorical, stable, and given—this option is
usually derisively dismissed—or, if we reject this picture, we can treat
it as a 'social construction' that is highly dynamic, assuming a new
form at each historical moment and reconstituted very recently in the
context of current technological, political, and representational inno-
vations.[2] For example, Margrit Shildrick claims that new reproductive
technologies vary the "space and boundaries between bodies" and
"dismantle old distinctions, supposedly guaranteed by a fixed biology." Such technologies, she claims, are "effectively postmodern in
their own right, [in their] refusal to accept the notion of an unchanging

natural body, and their capacity to problematize the grounds of (self) identity."[3] And Donna Haraway's highly influential "Cyborg Manifesto" celebrates and claims the breakdown of the stable boundaries around women's bodies and the overcoming of distinctions such as public/private, inside/outside, and nature/artifice, attributing this breakdown specifically to post-1980 developments in biotechnology and politics.[4]

But here, I have taken a less flashy middle path. I have worked to present the contemporary maternal body as neither timeless and given, nor a postmodern product of recent discourses, technologies, or institutions. The rejection of the "unchanging natural body" finds its ground not in postmodern feminism but in late Enlightenment Rousseauian sentimentalism. While the maternal body is a historical entity, the history of the maternal body is mostly one of robust continuities and endurance. Recent changes in the social and medical practices surrounding mothers' bodies have indeed produced changes in how those bodies are bounded, constituted, and gripped by norms, but it remains the case that the contemporary form of the maternal body is grounded in deeply *modern*—rather than postmodern—concerns, practices, and tensions.

Let us remind ourselves of some of these continuities. Since the Enlightenment, we have placed responsibility upon mothers' bodies for the formation of human nature, and through it the body politic. In assuming this responsibility, the maternal body became a juncture where medical and political concerns would continue to be mutually determining. We have treated pregnancy as an active project and the pregnant body as in need of self-discipline and as accountable to medical and social authorities for the operations of this discipline. The power of mothers' bodies to form and to deform has given us reason to regulate and monitor the boundaries and the workings of these bodies, and our civic investment in the products of these bodies has motivated us to displace their surface and their insides into public space. At the same time, we have taken mothers as properly and naturally sutured to their infants, the space and boundaries between them erased by the bond of milk. In imagination and practice, we have taken the boundaries of the maternal body as permeable, sometimes transparent, and always in need of protection, whether this is protection from the unruly and capricious appetites of the mother herself, or protection from the external forces that would separate and interrupt her naturally immaculate body.

I have argued that the figures of the Unruly and the Fetish Mother, which crystallized during the late eighteenth and early nineteenth centuries, continue to animate our contemporary understanding and care of maternal bodies. Both these figures are rooted in the shared idea that the maternal body, through its material practices and spatial arrangement, is the special seat of responsibility for the proper material and moral ordering of human nature. Both figures govern actual mothers' bodies most vividly through guiding the negotiation and arrangement of the spatial boundaries of these bodies: their policing, extension, reconfiguration, erasure, penetration, and representation. The late Enlightenment established a lasting tradition of taking the propriety of these boundaries as a linchpin of the proper ordering of human nature, and this tradition has persisted through shifts in our theoretical and practical beliefs about exactly how these boundaries should be configured.

Our fear of monsters, hybrids, and hysterics provides another common thread. Our old fear of Frankensteinian monsters and man-midwives has translated into an analogous fear of 'designer babies,' ectogenetic reproductive technologies, and the megalomaniacal scientists and unnatural mothers who are creating them. Our fear of wet nurses has translated into a fear of career and welfare moms wielding artificial nipples. We make the cut between so-called 'natural' childbirth and its complement ('unnatural' childbirth? 'artificial' childbirth?) as we did two centuries ago, on the basis of whether the skin of the maternal body is penetrated or punctured by an alien instrument. Massages and herbs are somehow deemed 'natural' whereas knives, needles, and forceps are not, and, without any particular grounding in empirical evidence concerning health outcomes, we continue to valorize the mother who proves her immaculate maternal status by completing childbirth without such interventions (even as, at the same time, we mark many maternal bodies as too riddled with risk—too old, too slow to dilate, too fat, too early, too late—to have the right to even attempt such a 'natural' birth). In laying claim to a cyborg identity, Haraway reclaims unruliness, hysteria, and the mixing of the 'natural' and the 'artificial' and thereby resists the normative tribunal of the Fetish Mother—"I would rather be a cyborg than a goddess."[5] Haraway's celebration of the cyborg is an empowering response to certain anxieties that are characteristically modern.

Recent technologies have allowed for an intensification and literalizing of the displacement of the fetus into public space and its transformation into a public figure. The externalized, public uterus—the source and symptom of our collective or mass hysteria—has become a robust part of the first-personal phenomenology of pregnancy through our enhanced capacity to represent fetuses and canonize pregnancy narratives. And recent intellectual and political movements have elevated one essential feature of the extended Fetish Mother, namely her *proximity* to her infant, emblematically through her breast, into a governing principle and figure of mothering. So there have been recent changes. But these are changes that strengthen or refocus dimensions of the ontology, science, politics, and phenomenology of embodied motherhood that have been spreading roots for at least a quarter of a millennium.

DECENTERED MOTHERS—UNFIXED BOUNDARIES

I have argued that the Fetish Mother and the Unruly Mother are bounded differently, both from one another and from 'normal' individual bodies. But I have tried to show that these two figures have a common origin and that they are complementary outgrowths of a single set of anxieties. Furthermore, as culturally live figures, they have importantly similar effects upon actual mothers' bodies. Both put the maternal body to work as a public and publicly owned figure and, correspondingly, divest mothers of certain basic rights to bodily privacy. Both require the subjection of some of the mother's bodily needs to the needs of the infant and the body politic. This can include her brute physical needs, for instance when she is expected to refrain from taking medications that she needs during pregnancy or to donate the iron in her blood and the calcium in her bones to her infant by breastfeeding under conditions of scarcity. But it also includes her somatic needs for privacy, separateness, space, and limitations on access to her body. Both are used to counter the fear that if women are granted bodily privacy and autonomy, they will become a chaotic and capricious deforming influence upon their children, wielding their autonomy as a weapon against their offspring. Both are represented in ways that render mothers anonymous: Images of the Fetish Mother are, as we saw, never images of particular women but rather of mythic icons, while images of public fetuses, displaced wombs, and canonical pregnancies require transparent and fungible maternal bodies. Most generally, both figures work to erase or puncture the boundaries around a mother's body that establish and incarnate her as a unified agent with integrity and autonomous agency.

During their pregnancies, contemporary North American women are for the most part treated as having unruly bodies—bodies rendered transparent so that their insides can be properly displaced, publicized, and disciplined in line with the common good. After they give birth, these same women are asked to give up their bodily boundaries once again, so as to form an extended romantic unity with the infant. There seems to be an ironic reversal going on here: We deny that the fetus is part of the woman's body while it is inside her and insist on the infant being part of her body once it is outside of her. During pregnancy, we treat the fetus as a primary and independent 'patient' or object of medical attention, and the mother's body becomes at best a medium of and at worst an obstacle to care for the fetus. Yet after birth we care for the 'maternal-child dyad' or the 'nursing couple.' Partly in an effort to control for what we have perceived as the ever-present potential for the mother's body to *turn against* its child—to provide a 'poison environment' during pregnancy and to separate and abandon the child after birth—we treat the fetus as in need of external protection during pregnancy, and we try to cement the mother and infant together and foreclose a boundary between them and around the mother after birth. In neither case does the mother herself emerge as a coherent focus of medical care and attention. (Indeed, even a woman's primary care fragments her in a way that men's does not; as many have noted, she goes to a general practitioner for care of those parts of her that do not concern reproduction and a gynecologist for care of those parts of her that do.)

One way in which the figures of the Fetish Mother and the Unruly Mother jointly undermine the integrity of the maternal self is by each giving social meanings and purposes to mothers' bodies that are essentially other-directed, where this other-directedness springs from the larger public function and responsibilities attributed to these bodies. Technologies and practices that elevate fetuses to independent patients will help to construe the mother's own body as an instrumental conduit for fetal outcomes. Breastfeeding literature is riddled with testimonies to women's supposed joy at discovering what their breasts are 'for.' Janet Tamaro's 1998 breastfeeding guide is in fact entitled *So That's What They're For!*[6] The title suggests that our breasts must have some essential meaning, and it is our job to discover (rather than establish) what this meaning is. In turn, this assumes that women do not manage to have a first-personal understanding of the 'point' of their bodies, except through the medium of the third-personal, other-involving functions of those bodies. In much breastfeeding literature, reading our breasts as 'for' breastfeeding is portrayed as liberating insofar as it allows us to resist reading them as 'for' the erotic male gaze. This disjunction was explicit during a 1984 rally against the media exploitation of women's bodies, where women marched topless and carried placards reading, "Our breasts are *for the newborn*, not for men's porn."[7] But it is unfortunate if we can only resist defining our bodies in terms of male desire by defining them in terms of infant desire, without challenging the idea that the meanings of our body parts are publicly established and other-directed.

Contemporary labor and birth (which have commanded much less of my attention, in this book, than pregnancy and early motherhood) are situated within cultural and medical institutions in ways that vividly exemplify the interplay between our fetishization of proximity and 'natural' maternality, on the one hand, and our desire to control for unruly and capricious maternal behavior through external interventions, on the other. For example, "progressive" hospitals now place a heavy emphasis on the 'bonding' that is supposed to occur between mothers and infants in the first few days or even minutes after their birth. To further this bonding, new mothers, including those who have had cesarean sections, are encouraged to see and hold their babies right after birth and are expected to breastfeed within an hour of the birth; afterward the 'good' mother will enthusiastically acquiesce to the proud hospital's offer to let the baby share her room rather than sleep in the nursery (thereby voluntarily giving up her last chance for a good night's sleep for the next few months at least). On the whole, these practices manifest obvious improvements over the days when women were routinely put under general anesthetic for the birth, and infants were whisked away to the nursery to receive bottles and be cooed at from behind glass. On the other hand, the stress on the supposedly pivotal importance of these initial moments of contact to the whole mother-child relationship continues the fetishization of mute proximity that we examined in chapter 5. Furthermore, our concern with mothers' 'bonding' with their children during the first few hours is premised on the idea that they need to cross a divide that separates them, and this divide is of course institutionalized in the practices during pregnancy and labor that displace the fetus away from the body and into independent, public space. Moreover, these normatively loaded practices plant a few fetishized moments of mandatory proximity in the midst of a birth process that has been largely taken out of mothers' hands. Our standard birth practices embed the suggestion that the bond between mother and child can be created and cemented through rituals of nearness contained in the period right after birth, regardless of how alienating we make the environment surrounding these rituals.

The 'natural childbirth' invokes the fetishistic language of nature to give some laboring and mothering practices a *moral* value in virtue of their maintenance of proximity and their freedom from alien penetrations. It treats 'natural' childbirth as somehow a more admirable accomplishment than 'medicalized' childbirth. It is important to notice that despite its nominal desire to bring the focus in obstetrical care back onto the woman, the normative weight attached to having a 'natural' birth, in this movement, is neither based on well-established risk and outcome measures (a charge equally leveled against those advocating standard medicalized hospital births), *nor* on a particular woman's sense of what is valuable to her and makes her comfortable during childbirth and pregnancy—an authentic choice against 'nature' is simply not an option for mothers in the moral ontology of the natural childbirth movement.[8] In protecting the mother from artificial interventions, the natural childbirth movement suggests that the quality of her mothering is at stake in this protection and that something as simple as an epidural needle could corrupt her maternality and render her unruly.

Even if we could make some sense of the idea that some birth and mothering practices are "more natural" than others, we need to remember that even the most "natural" maternal practices occur in a cultural context in which pregnancy, labor, and mothering are regulated, disciplined, and monitored at every stage. The breastfeeding mother who smugly made it through a vaginal delivery without an epidural is still very unlikely to have escaped the constitutive influence of pregnancy manuals, web calendars, dietary regimes, and the like. We choose a few fetishized moments—the actual exit of the infant from the mother's body, infant feeding practices—and elevate them into the markers of proper 'natural' mothering. Mothers who *choose* pain medications, hospital births, and even cesarean sections are demonized as unmaternal cyborg hysterics who have, through their choices about how to manage twelve or twenty-four hours of labor, already set the stage for a lifetime of separation and antagonism between themselves and their children.

Thus both standard 'medicalized' birth practices and 'natural' birth practices, as institutions, encode both a fetishization of natural proximity and a fear of the capacity of the maternal body to be unruly, and neither challenge traditional notions of maternal 'nature' or of the supposed fragility of women's capacity to mother well. These institutions resist one another from two sides of the same ideological coin and thereby in effect reinforce one another's presuppositions. The *medicalization* of pregnancy, birth, and mothering is not, in and of itself, what renders these processes alienating, violating, and self-erasing for many women. In fact, as I argued in chapter 1, early attempts to bring reproductive health into the domain of medical discourse were if anything motivated by a proto-feminist (though double-edged) desire to demarginalize and humanize women's health. Rather, the threats to mothers' embodied self devolve, I would claim, from our social and medical refusal to grant their boundaries the same solidity and their domain of privacy the same integrity as those of other citizens. In this refusal, contemporary versions of medical interventionism and the rhetoric of the 'natural' equally collude.

SOLIDIFYING THE MATERNAL SELF

As feminists, we can respond in various ways to the boundary violations, reconfigurations, and co-options that have marked the history of the maternal body. One strategy is to claim the shifting, permeable, expandable, unresolvable boundaries of the feminine and/or maternal body[9] as a positive identity. This strand of feminist thought begins with the recognition of how women's and especially mothers' bodies have been configured in contrast to the traditionally bounded, static, impermeable masculine body,[10] and it seeks to empower women through this very contrast, accepting the characterization but rejecting or reversing its normative force. Thus Patrice DiQuinzio, in *The Impossibility of Motherhood*,[11] wants a theory of subjectivity that makes it "partial, divided and fragmented," and Margrit Shildrick, in *Leaky Bodies and Boundaries*, is dismissive of the "humanist presupposition of an integrated subjectivity," insisting on "instability" and "above all leakiness as the very ground for a post modern feminist ethic." For her, "the deconstruction of boundaries . . . is at the heart of the postmodernist feminist enterprise," and bodily boundaries are her primary target.[12] Theorists such as Donna Haraway and Elizabeth Grosz have reclaimed the failure of distinctions between self and other, inside and outside, whole and part that have historically been read as deficits in maternal or feminine subjectivity and bodies: "The cyborg is a kind of disassembled and reassembled, postmodern collective and personal self. This is the self feminists must code."[13]

French feminists in particular have defended the leaky, mutable, uncountable, overflowing female and maternal body as a critical source for new thought and writing and as a crucial seat of libratory politics. In her influential manifesto "The Laugh of the Medusa," Hélène Cixous ties femininity tightly to maternality and aligns the maternal body with a lack of separateness, claiming "A woman is never far from 'mother.'. . . There is always within her at least a little of that good mother's milk. She writes with white ink. . . . In women there is always more or less of the mother who makes everything all right, who nourishes, and who *stands up against separation*."[14] Thus

Cixous embraces the lack of a sharp and stable boundary around the body of the mother, siding with a lineage from Rousseau to La Leche League in positively valuing the bond of milk as the basis for an active refusal of separation between mother and infant, and by extension woman/mother and nourished nation. But she also embraces the boundary failures that have been associated with the Unruly Mother— the body prone to disorderly excess and leakage: "We're stormy, and that which is ours breaks loose from us without our fearing any debilitation. Our glances, our smiles, are spent; laughs exude from all our mouths, our blood flows and we extend ourselves without ever reaching an end."[15] Whereas historically, as we have seen, the extension of maternal boundaries to include the infant has been fetishized and valued, and the permeability and capriciousness of these boundaries have been feared and disciplined, Cixous embraces the elasticity and spatial perplexity of the maternal bodies in all their forms. Michelle Walker comments that Cixous is one of many feminists for whom "the maternal body is the emblem of a fluid and mutable identity."[16]

Equally exalted French feminist diva Luce Irigaray has participated in the fetishization of proximity and embraced the apparent capacity of the female/maternal body[17] to be unindividuatable, both one and two at once. In *This Sex Which Is Not One*, she writes,

> Woman always remains several, but she is kept from dispersion because the other is already within her and is autoerotically familiar to her. Which is not to say that she appropriates the other for herself, that she reduces it to her own property. Ownership and property are doubtless quite foreign to the feminine. At least sexually. But not *nearness*. Nearness so pronounced that it makes all discrimination of identity, and thus all forms of property, impossible. Woman derives pleasure from what is *so near that she cannot have it, nor have herself*. She herself enters into a ceaseless exchange of herself with the other without any possibility of identifying either.[18]

It seems to me that we cannot fail to recognize that there is something empowering in Irigaray's jubilant exhibition of the odd logic of feminine/maternal bodily space. I want to acknowledge a libratory dimension to such joyous and defiant embrace of the apparent tensions that the maternal body has born. I see an important theoretical and political place for writing that refuses to take the leaky, disorderly, extendable, unstable body as the *defective* or *problematic* counterpart to some mythical well-bounded, impenetrable, static masculine body. The exuberantly excessive body that acknowledges its ideological history and refuses to be shackled by it cuts an attractive figure indeed.

But in the end, I am deeply wary of these feminist reclaimings of the openness, fluidity, fragmentation, instability, and extendibility of maternal boundaries. Deconstructions of the distinction between self and other, however theoretically tempting, have proved problematic in the material life of mothers. A serious limitation of these reclaimings is that they cannot address the ways in which existing power structures are poised to co-opt a female body that does not own itself and whose boundaries and unity are in question. Women's bodies are vulnerable, and mothers' bodies particularly so. As I have stressed, social institutions have a strong and historically entrenched vested interest in violating the boundaries of such bodies, submitting them to public regulation and control, investing them with public meanings that co-opt their semiotics, and robbing them of their right to various important kinds of privacy and separation. If the denigration of the unstable, excessive, permeable body had its life purely within an intellectual domain, then it might well be high time to resist this denigration through reveling in just those dimensions of our bodies that have been devalued. But I have tried to show here that while there are important intellectual roots to these ideologies of the body, in fact they have played themselves out in uncompromisingly concrete terms, shaping and often violating mothers' practical autonomy and safety. While authors such as Haraway and Irigaray are vividly aware of the history of exploitation of the nontraditional boundaries of maternal and feminine subjects, their reclaiming moves do not acknowledge the *practical* importance of being able to set firm boundaries when we need them, nor do they help mothers establish or ensure a stable body and agency strong enough to resist boundary crossings that are violating rather than liberating.

The sexual abuse survivor who experiences breastfeeding as an assault, the working mother who feels she has selfishly abandoned her infant if she allows another caregiver to give it a bottle during the day, the expectant woman who looks to the ultrasound monitor to be told the moral meaning of her pregnancy, and the pregnant woman who is scared to take antidepressants that pose only a theoretical risk to her fetus because she is held captive by an image of her risky and permeable womb will not be helped to restore appropriate boundaries and healthy integrity by the postmodern efforts to valorize the fragmented and permeable self. These are women whose difficulty is not intellectual—they do not suffer, as philosophical writing often does, from being held captive by underconstructed seventeenth-century Hobbesian and Cartesian models of self-contained subjectivity. Practically speaking, we need a strongly cohesive self with healthy and robust boundaries before we can care well for ourselves or for others. Jane Flax, drawing upon her experience as a practicing therapist, warns, "Those who celebrate or call for a 'decentered' self seem self-deceptively naïve and unaware of the basic cohesion within themselves that makes the fragmentation of experiences something other than a terrifying slide into psychosis."[19]

Cautioning feminists who rush to sign onto the postmodern deconstruction and fragmentation of subjectivity, Nancy Hartsock asks us to wonder, "Why is it that just at the moment when so many of us who have been silenced begin to demand the right to name ourselves, to act as subjects rather than objects of history, that just then the concept of subjecthood becomes problematic?"[20] Similarly, as feminists, I think we need to be very cautious before riding the postmodern wave of body deconstruction. Margrit Shildrick, responding to Hartsock, counters that the crisis of modernity is a male crisis because women were never accorded the stable subjectivity that postmodern critiques put into question. Thus, she concludes, feminists have nothing to lose, as it were, and should not be afraid to embrace these critiques.[21] But at least in the domain of the body, I have been trying to show that the fragmentation, permeation, public co-option, and uncertain individuation of mothers' bodies have in many ways constituted a crisis *for women*, materially and emotionally if not intellectually. The body that is marked by strong boundaries, a distinction between inner and outer, self and other, and private and public, is a currently fashionable target of theoretical disdain and postmodern play. But it may well be that such subversive play is a privilege of those bodies that can safely support the self through it because they already have the necessary freedom of movement, freedom from vulnerability, and stability of identity. Once the boundaries of our bodies are secure and we can navigate and protect our own private and public spaces, then we may be able to play with these boundaries and spaces from a position of safety and strength.

Consider the private/public distinction, once a staple of political theory, which has for quite a while come under eloquent attack by feminist and postmodernist theorists. Classical political thought divided human life into private domestic space, in which women were supposed to be contained, and public, civic space, marked as masculine or at least by the absence of the feminine. Twentieth-century liberal theory, including liberal feminist theory, worked to extend and refine this basic distinction by defining the body itself as a private space within which the state had no place. At roughly the same time as the supreme court of the United States decided (in *Roe v. Wade*) that women's freedom of reproductive choice was constitutionally protected specifically in virtue of the *privacy* of the body, Canadian Prime Minister Pierre Trudeau struck all references to homosexuality out of the criminal code, famously declaring on national television that "the state has no business in the bedrooms of the nation." The goal, for liberal feminists, was not to overthrow the private/public distinction, but to enhance it, while at the same time giving both men and women equal access to both domains. But as their feminist daughters developed the insight that "the personal is political," and the boundaries between private and public space revealed themselves to be inherently context-bound, interpenetrated, and likely incoherent, postmodernists quickly heralded the death of the private/public distinction itself.

But while political theory is much richer and subtler for having recognized that this distinction will never be stable or clean, this doesn't mean that we can safely obliterate it, and current threats to its constitutional protection in the United States only make this all the more clear. The fact is that while women have traditionally been read as contained in the 'private domain,' mothering is a practice and a responsibility that clearly exceeds this containment. Hegel (anachronistically) attributes to Sophocles the insight that mothers, in creating public citizens who will leave the private domain, do private work that is inherently public in its meaning,[22] and we have seen that mothers' bodies have long been used as crucial public spectacles. Mothers' most private body parts and behaviors have public significance, and, as Linda Blum puts it, the maternal body "always has obligations to the larger social body. . . . [M]otherhood and breastfeeding are and continue to be public matters."[23] While it is empowering to acknowledge this inherent publicity, in order to counter a privacy that has been associated with shame and confined domesticity, there are other kinds of privacy we cannot relinquish—not all of our practices and body parts can be available for public scrutiny, public co-option of meaning, or public accountability.

Throughout the second half of this book, I tried to show that mothers are socially, materially, and imaginatively positioned in ways that make it difficult for them to understand, negotiate, and protect their own bodily and phenomenological boundaries. Yet our safe and healthy embodied selfhood requires spaces of privacy and publicity that we can move into and out of as needed and boundaries whose opening and closing is substantially under our own control. Feminists have been very clear about how crucial these bodily needs are in the domain of sexuality, but we have attended much less to how pregnancy, labor, and early motherhood also require the negotiation of bodily space and boundaries. Indeed, women can face vulnerabilities and challenges to their identity in the maternal domain that are deeply analogous to and even overlap with those they face in the sexual domain.

Postmodernists are surely right that the various binary distinctions that have historically been used to mark out bodies and subjects are not stable or metaphysically given. Inner and outer, private and public, self and other are domains that are constituted in and through social, material, and intellectual practices, and the boundaries between them are in many ways the products of our social interactions and representations rather than their origin and ground. Indeed, I have been examining this process of production throughout this book. In my view, the great insight and power of postmodernism is to reveal how its modernist predecessors *fetishized* such distinctions. That is, historically, we treated these distinctions as, on the one hand, ahistorical and 'naturally' given and, on the other hand, as intrinsically normative, capable of grounding value judgments.[24] In theory and in practice, we have treated the failure and flexibility of mothers' boundaries as a fixed fact that explains rather than is explained by social forces, and we have used certain pictures of masculine and feminine bodies as tribunals of the natural and the appropriate. Recent theorists are absolutely right about two things: these naturalizing and fetishizing moves are ideological maneuvers based on an incorrect metaphysics, and these moves need to be critiqued and revealed as the weapons of ideology that they are.

However, the revelation that a distinction is historically shifting, ideologically motivated, politically potent, and constituted through social and material practice should *in no way* be taken as evidence that the distinction is not real or important to preserve. We can recognize the need to defetishize and critically interrogate a distinction even while we fight to maintain it. We need to pursue a rigorous theoretical examination and critique of the naturalizing moves that make these marks, boundaries, and distinctions look simply given rather than earned, but this examination should support rather than detract from our efforts to go ahead and earn them for ourselves. Such distinctions and boundaries are *accomplishments* and not metaphysical givens.

In insisting on creating social conditions in which mothers can have well-bounded and coherent selves, protection from unwanted penetration, private and public space, and the freedom to move between them both with and without their children, we should not simply work to establish or reinstate the so-called traditional 'liberal' self.

For this liberal self defines and establishes its boundaries and its domain of privacy in a historically specific way that has been uncomfortable for feminists, and with good reason. Traditionally, the liberal self does not just have boundaries that establish it as *separate from* others; rather, its boundaries, of their very essence, make it *independent* of others, even *antagonistic* toward others. The practical agency of the classical liberal self is defined in terms of a self-contained will and set of interests that can be understood as fully independent of and prior to the wills and interests of others. Analogously, liberal privacy has been an inherently *exclusionary* notion; the right to privacy has been interpreted as the right to total dominion or sovereignty over one's body and domestic space—the right and the ability to quite literally "keep it to oneself." The ontology of the liberal self sets up a logic in which relationships between two people can only be understood in two ways, as either "conflicting" or "unified": we are either in presumptive conflict with one another because we are separate people and our interests and will have nothing essential to do with one another, or we must be 'one with' each other, in effect the same person as that other. This opposition was a deeply embedded starting point for Rousseau's thought, as we saw in chapter 2. According to him, the only way that we could be anything other than fully independent centers of will and value with no hope of supporting one another's ends except through contingent coincidence was if we could be constructed as creatures with a single identity and a single general will. It was out of this dichotomy between total separation and total identity that his tasks for the maternal body were born in the first place.

Now I think that much of the feminist urge to sign onto postmodernist deconstructions of the well-bounded self has in fact come from a very reasonable discomfort with this set of liberal options and oppositions, combined with the false assumption that rejecting them must involve rejecting wholesale the ideals of cohesive agency, boundaries, and identifiable distinctions between private and public domains. Shildrick makes this link explicit: "To . . . insist on and defend the unity and closure of the maternal subject can *only* collude with the phallocratic insistence on identity as that which excludes the other."[25] Elsewhere she equates the "security of the material boundaries of the body" with the "exclusion of otherness."[26] But this is to allow the models of selfhood we want to reject define the terms of the debate. I see every reason not to concede to these equations, which are inadequate to mothers' experiences and needs.

To assume that the protection of boundaries and privacy is a protection of radical independence and exclusion is to assume that the self that seeks boundaries and privacy is a self who will find integrity and self-definition through the abandonment of intimate relationships and through the pitting of her interests against those of her children. It is this assumption that has led much medical and bioethical discourse to cast any issue in which pregnant women and their future children must be considered *separately* as one of "maternal-fetal conflict." It allowed Judith Jarvis Thompson to imagine pregnancy as an artificial tube connecting us to a stranger who limits our freedom and drains our bodily resources.[27]

We mothers are neither simply 'one with' our children, nor simply independent of them; assimilation and abandonment are not our only options. We have inherited a model of selfhood, from Rousseau and other humanists, that can easily foreclose our ability to articulate other possibilities and be heard. But we can and usually do have deep, self-defining, intimate relationships with our children that do not erase the boundaries between us. What mothers strive for, when we strive to set boundaries, is almost never complete dominion over our bodies and spaces. Nor do we seek to forge interests and life plans that exclude our children. When we seek integrity, well-established boundaries, protection against vulnerabilities, and the right to privacy, we overwhelmingly do so as individuals who are utterly and self-definingly invested in our children's flourishing, reeling from our love for them, incapable of even thinking the possibility of abandonment. The fact that our children shape the very terrain of our life possibilities—where we would consider living, what jobs we would consider taking, what relationships with other family members we are determined to sustain—is usually cause for our commitment and celebration, not selfish or grudging regret. None of this detracts *in the slightest* from our very real need for limits, privacy, a separate identity, self-determination, and a room of our own. Nor does it detract from our need to have a basic (though realistic) level of trust in our bodies, nor from our need to be cared for by social and medical institutions as whole individuals with integrity, as opposed to either capricious appetite-machines and fragmented conduits of deformation, or idealized, fetishized creatures of nature. A strong and separate sense of self, protection from bodily violations and vulnerabilities, and access to our own social and medical care empower us to act well on our maternal love rather than call it into question.

In short, then, I think that as theoretically fraught as the terms may be, there are crucial pragmatic and political reasons to insist upon the boundaries of our bodies and on robust distinctions between public and private space. At the same time, though, we need to reveal the historicity, the vulnerability, and the contingency of these boundaries and distinctions, and we need to resist every equation of boundaries and privacy with exclusion, abandonment, and antagonism. Women (like men) are indeed leaky and permeable, and our boundaries are complex and shifting. Our need to continuously *negotiate* the boundaries between others and ourselves shows that these boundaries are not given or absolute. But these facts call for the ongoing establishment and resolution of boundaries, not their erasure or fragmentation. Only once mothers have access to secure and appropriate boundaries will it be safe to engage in the kind of carefree boundary-play that Irigaray, Cixous, Shildrick, Haraway, and others so alluringly inscribe.

I have tried to reveal a centuries-old history during which mothers' bodily boundaries have been opened, expanded, reconfigured, erased, and distrusted by various constellations of scientific, social, and representational practices. I have argued for the need to affirm and 'fix' these boundaries, separating inside from outside, private from public, and self from other. The fact that our projects and identities are often ineliminably bound to our caring commitment to the flourishing of our actual and future children does not pose a threat to these boundaries. On the other hand, the displacement and co-option of the insides of our bodies, our being treated instrumentally and partially at the hands of social and medical institutions, and the social challenges that greet us when we seek to separate and protect ourselves do constitute assaults on these boundaries. We need to *fix* our boundaries in at least three senses: we need to *repair* them, we need to *settle* them (though always provisionally and with flexibility), and we need to *reclaim* their meanings from those who would interpret any quest for boundaries as a compromise of our maternality.

NOTES

1. Foucault (New York: Vintage Books, 1984), 199.
2. This is the explicit thesis of Karen Newman, *Fetal Positions* (Palo Alto: Stanford University Press, 1996).
3. Shildrick, *Leaky Bodies and Boundaries* (New York: Routledge, 1997), 180–81.
4. "The Cyborg Manifesto," in Haraway, *Simians, Cyborgs and Women: The Reinvention of Nature* (New York: Routlege, 1991). For other works that read the maternal body as radically reconfigured by very recent technological and institutional changes, see chapter 1, footnote 14 above.
5. Haraway 1991, 181.
6. Tamaro (Holbrook, MA: Adams Media Corp., 1998).
7. Reported in Miriam Yalom, *A Short History of the Breast* (New York: Ballantine Books, 1997), my emphasis.

8. For example, Al-Yasha Ilhaam Williams and Ina May Gaskin describe the choice to receive medical interventions during birth, particularly a cesarean section, as an 'empty' choice; indeed, calling it a choice at all, they claim, "constitutes an appropriation of feminist language without feminist political content." "Elective Cesareans as Reproductive Choice: Some Ethical Considerations," unpublished manuscript, 2004.

9. I should note that with disjunctive expressions such as this, I by no means wish to conflate feminine and maternal subjectivity. I bring the terms together here only because amongst the theorists who make the kind of reclaiming move I am examining here, some target maternal bodies and subjectivity, others target feminine bodies and subjectivity more generally, and others do not draw as much distinction between the two as we might wish for.

10. This version of the masculine body is a fetish, just as is the body of the Fetish Mother. Actual men of course experience boundary violations, permeations, and other instabilities. But masculinity, it is easy to argue, has been normatively governed by this fetish ideal of solidity and impermeability, just as maternality has been governed by fetish ideals of extended unity.

11. New York: Routledge, 1999.

12. Shildrick 1997, 156, 12, 2.

13. Haraway 1991, 163. See also Elizabeth Grosz, *Volatile Bodies* (New York: Routledge, 1999).

14. "The Laugh of the Medusa," trans. K. Cohen and P. Cohen, *Signs: Journal of Women in Culture and Society* 1(4), 1976, 875–93, 881–82.

15. Cixous 1976, 878.

16. Walker, *Philosophy and the Maternal Body: Reading Silence* (New York: Routledge, 1998), 139.

17. Unlike Cixous, Irigaray resists taking the maternal body as the simple essence of the feminine body, and instead she figures the feminine body via its sexuality. However, it is no accident that the language she uses to inscribe the sexual feminine body borrows the metaphors and imagery of pregnancy and birth.

18. Irigaray, *This Sex Which Is Not One*, trans. C. Porter (Ithaca: Cornell University Press, 1995), 31. Emphasis in the original.

19. Flax, *Thinking Fragments: Psychoanalysis, Feminism, Postmodernism in the Contemporary West* (Berkeley: University of California Press, 1990), 218–19.

20. Hartsock, "Foucault on Power: A Theory for Women," in Linda Nicholson, *Feminism/Postmodernism* (New York: Routledge, 1989).

21. Shildrick 1997, 144–45.

22. See Hegel's reading of *Antigone* in the *Phenomenology of Sprit*, trans. A. V. Miller (New York: Oxford University Press, 1977).

23. Blum, *At the Breast* (Boston: Beacon Press, 1999), 2.

24. See my discussion of fetishization in chapter 3.

25. Shildrick 1997, 208, my emphasis.

26. Shildrick 1997, 11.

27. Judith Jarvis Thompson, "A Defense of Abortion," *Philosophy and Public Affairs* 1(1), 1971, 47–66.

Bibliography

Abbott, John. *The Mother at Home, or the Principles of Maternal Duty*. Boston: Crocker and Brewster, 1833.

Althusser, L. "Ideology and Ideological State Apparatuses," in *Lenin and Philosophy*. London: New Left Books, 1971.

Andrews, Lori B. *The Clone Age: Adventures in the New World of Reproductive Technology*. New York: Holt, 1999.

American Academy of Pediatrics. "Breastfeeding and the Use of Human Milk: Policy Statement," *Pediatrics* 100 no. 6, 1997: 1035–39.

American Academy of Pediatrics. *New Mother's Guide to Breastfeeding*. New York: Bantam, 2002.

Anonymous. *The English Midwife Enlarged*. London: Rowland Reynolds, 1682.

Anonymous. *Aristotle's Masterpiece, or the Secret of Generation Displayed in all the Parts Thereof*. London 1684.

Anonymous. *An Important Address to Wives and Mothers on the Dangers and Immorality of Man-Midwifery*. London: Lewis and Co., 1830.

Armstrong, Elizabeth M. *Conceiving Risk, Bearing Responsibility: Fetal Alcohol Syndrome and the Diagnosis of Moral Disorder*. Baltimore: Johns Hopkins University Press, 2003.

Asquith, M. T., et al. "The Bacterial Content of Breast Milk after the Early Initiation of Expression Using a Standard Technique," *Journal of Pediatric Gastroenterology and Nutrition* 3 no. 1, 1984: 104–7.

Avery, M. D., L. Duckett and C. R. Frantzich. "The Experience of Sexuality During Breastfeeding Among Primiparous Women," *Journal of Midwifery and Women's Health* 45 no. 3, 2000: 227–37.

Barad, Karen. "Getting Real: Technoscientific Practices and the Materialization of Reality," *Differences* 10, no. 2. 1998: 86–128.

Bard, Samuel. *A Compendium of the Theory and Practice of Midwifery*. New York: Collins and Co., 1817.

Barnes, J., et al. "Extreme Attitudes to Body Shape, Social and Psychological Factors, and a Reluctance to Breast Feed," *Journal of the Royal Society of Medicine* 90 no. 10, 1997: 551–59.

Bauer, Ingrid. "Natural Infant Hygiene: A Gentle Alternative to Long-Term Diapering," at www.natural-wisdom.com/nihgentlealternative.htm, accessed June 2005.

Bellamy, E. "Mother Love Gone Wrong," *The Weekend Australian Review*, March 21 1998: 16–17.

Bentham, Jeremy. *The Panopticon Writings*, edited by M. Bozovic. New York: Verso, 1995.

Bianchini, Giovanni. *Essay on the Force of the Imagination in Pregnant Women*. London, trans. 1772.

Billout, M. F. *Dissertation sur l'Hygiene des Femmes Encients*. Paris: Didot Jeune, 1816.

Blondel, James. *The Force of the Mother's Imagination upon her Foetus in Utero*. London: J. Walthoe, 1730.

Blum, Carol. *Rousseau and the Republic of Virtue*. Ithaca: Cornell University Press, 1986.

Blum, Linda. *At the Breast: Ideologies of Breastfeeding and Motherhood in the Contemporary United States*. Boston: Beacon Press, 1999.

Blundell, James. *The Principles and Practice of Obstetrics as at Present Taught*. Washington: Duff Green, 1834.

Blunt, John. *Man-Midwifery Dissected*. London: S. W. Fores, 1793.

Bobel, Chris. *The Paradox of Natural Mothering*. Philadelphia: Temple University Press, 2002.

Bordo, Susan. *Unbearable Weight: Feminism, Western Culture and the Body*. Berkeley: University of California Press, 1995.

Bourne, Gordon L. *Pregnancy*. New York: Harper and Row, 1975.

Brown, Amy B. and McPherson, Kathryn, editors. *The Reality of Breastfeeding: Reflections by Contemporary Women*. New York: Bergin and Garvey, 1998.

Buchan, William. *Advice to Mothers on the Subject of Their Own Health, and of the Means of Promoting the Health, Strength and Beauty of Their Offspring*. Boston: J. Bumstead, 1809.

Burby, Leslie, for "ProMoM." "101 Reasons to Breastfeed Your Child," www .promom.org/101/index.html, accessed June 2005.

Bull, Thomas. *Hints to Mothers, for the Management of Health During the Period of Pregnancy, and in the Lying-In Room*. New York: J. Wiley, 1842.

Burns, James. *Principles of Midwifery*. New York: Joseph H. Francis, 1837.

Cadogan, William. *Essay upon Nursing and the Management of Children from Birth to Three Years of Age*, London, J. Roberts, 1748, reprinted in M. and J. Rendle-Short, *The Father of Child Care*. Bristol: John Wright and Sons, 1966.

Carter, Pam. *Feminism, Breasts and Breastfeeding*. New York: Palgrave MacMillan, 1995.

Cazeaux, P. *A Theoretical and Practical Treatise on Midwifery, Including the Diseases of Pregnancy and Parturition*, translated by R. P. Thomas. Philadelphia: Lindsay and Blakiston, 1805.

Chavasse, P. H., *The Physical Training of Children*. Philadelphia: New World Publishing 1872.

Churchill, Fleetwood. *On the Diseases of Women; Including Those of Pregnancy and Childbirth*. Philadelphia: Blanchard and Lea, 1857.

Churchill, Fleetwood. *On the Theory and Practice of Midwifery*. Philadelphia: Blanchard and Lea, 1860.

Cixous, Hélène. "The Laugh of the Medusa," translated by K. Cohen and P. Cohen, *Signs: Journal of Women in Culture and Society* 1 no. 4, 1976: 875–93.

Coleman, A. and L. Coleman. "Completing the Female Sexual Cycle: Intercourse, Childbirth and Breastfeeding," *Sexual Medicine Today* 2 no. 5, 1978: 34–40.

Coles, Walter. *The Nurse and Mother: A Manual for the Guidance of Monthly Nurses and Mothers*. Chicago: J. H. Chambers and Co., 1881.

Colin, W. B. and J. A. Scott. "Breastfeeding: Reasons for Starting, Reasons for Stopping, and Problems Along the Way," *Breastfeeding Review* 10 no. 2, 2002: 13–19.

Conde-Agudelo, A., J. L. Diaz-Rossell, and J. L. Belizan. "Kangaroo Mother Care to Reduce Morbidity and Mortality in Low Birthweight Infants," *Birth* 30 no. 2, 2003: 133–34.

Cronenwett, L. et al. "Single Daily Bottle Use in the Early Weeks Post-Partum and Breastfeeding Outcomes," *Pediatrics* 90 no. 5, 1992: 760–66.

Culpeper, Nicholas. *Directory for Midwives.* London: Peter Cole, 1656.

Davis-Floyd, Robbie, and Joseph Dumit, editors. *Cyborg Babies: From Techno-Sex to Techno-Tots.* New York: Routledge, 1998.

Dettwyler, K. "Beauty and the Breast," in *Breastfeeding: Biocultural Perspectives,* edited by P. Stuart-MacAdam and K. A. Dettwyler. New York: De Gruyter, 1995.

Deutsche, Helen. *The Psychology of Women,* Volume 2. New York: Grune and Stratton, 1945.

Digman, Denise M. "Understanding Intimacy as Experienced by Breastfeeding Mothers," *Health Care for Women International* 16 no. 5, 1995: 477–85.

DiQuinzio, Patrice. *The Impossibility of Motherhood.* New York: Routledge, 1999.

Dionis, Pierre. *A General Treatise on Midwifery.* London: A. Bell, trans. 1719.

Doane, Janice and Devon Hodges. *From Klein to Kristeva: Psychoanalytic Feminism and the Search for the 'Good-Enough' Mother.* Ann Arbor: University of Michigan Press, 1992.

Donné, Alfred. *Mothers and Infants, Nurses and Nursing.* Boston: Phillips, Spapson and Co., trans. 1859.

Dreyfus, Hubert. *What Computers Cannot Do.* New York: Harper Collins 1979.

Dreyfus, Hubert. *Being-in-the-World: A Commentary on Heidegger's "Being and Time" Division I.* Cambridge, MA: MIT Press, 1990.

Duden, Barbara. *Disembodying Woman: Perspectives on Pregnancy and the Unborn,* translated by L. Hoinacki. Cambridge: Harvard University Press, 1993.

Duden, Barbara. *The Woman Beneath The Skin: A Doctor's Patients in Eighteenth-Century Germany,* translated by T. Dunlap. Cambridge: Harvard University Press, 1997.

Eagleton, Terry. *The Ideology of the Aesthetic.* New York: Blackwell, 1990.

Eisenberg, A., H. Murkoff and S. Hathaway. *What to Expect in the First Year.* New York: Workman Publishing, 1989.

Eisenberg, A., H. Murkoff and S. Hathaway. *What to Expect When You're Expecting Pregnancy Organizer.* New York: Workman Publishing, 1995.

Elkinton, John. *The Poison Womb: Human Reproduction in a Polluted World.* New York: Penguin, 1985.

Farr, Samuel. *Elements Of Medical Jurisprudence; Or A Succinct And Compendious Description Of Such Tokens In The Human Body As Are Requisite To Determine The Judgment Of A Coroner, And Courts Of Law, In Cases Of Divorce, Rape, Murder &C. To Which Are Added, Directions For Preserving The Public Health.* London: Callow, 1815.

Feldman, R., et al. "Testing a Family Intervention Hypothesis: The Contribution of Mother-Infant Skin-to-Skin Contact (Kangaroo Care) to Family Interaction, Proximity, and Touch," *Journal of Family Psychology* 17 no. 1, 2003: 94–107.

Feldman, Susan. "From Occupied Bodies to Pregnant Persons," in *Autonomy and Community: Readings in Contemporary Kantian Social Philosophy,* edited by J. Kneller and S. Axinn. Albany: SUNY Press, 1998.

Flax, Jane. *Thinking Fragments: Psychoanalysis, Feminism, Postmodernism in the Contemporary West.* Berkeley: University of California Press, 1990.

Foster, S. F., P. Slade and K. Wilson. "Body Image, Maternal Fetal Attachment and Breast-Feeding," *Journal of Psychosomatic Research* 41 no. 2, 1996: 181–84.

Fergusson, D. M. and L. J. Woodward. "Breastfeeding and Later Psychosocial Adjustment," *Paediatric and Perinatal Epidemiology* 12 no. 2, 1999: 144–57.

Fermon, Nicole. *Domesticating Passions: Rousseau, Woman and the Nation.* Hanover, NH: Wesleyan University Press, 1997.

Fisher, C. and S. Inch. "Nipple Confusion: Who Is Confused?" *Journal of Pediatrics* 129 no. 1, 1996: 174–75.

Fildes, Valerie. *Breasts, Bottles and Babies: A History of Infant Feeding.* Edinburgh: Edinburgh University Press, 1986.

Fissel, Mary. "Hairy Women and Naked Truths: Gender and the Politics of Knowledge in *Aristotle's Masterpiece,*" *The William and Mary Quarterly* 60 no. 1, 2003.

Fissel, Mary. "When the Womb Went Bad: Motherhood in Sixteenth Century England," in her *Vernacular Bodies: The Politics of Reproduction in Early Modern England.* New York: Cambridge University Press, 2004.

Fletcher, J. C. and M. I. Evans. "Maternal Bonding in Early Fetal Ultrasound Examinations," *New England Journal of Medicine* 308 no. 7, 1983: 382–83.

Foucault, Michel. *Discipline and Punish: The Birth of the Prison.* New York: Pantheon, 1977.

Foucault, Michel. *The Birth of the Clinic: An Archaeology of Medical Perception.* New York: Vintage Books, 1984.

Fowler, O. S. *Maternity: Or the Bearing and Nursing of Children, Including Female Education and Beauty.* New York: Fowler and Wells, 1856.

Georges, Eugenia and Lisa M. Mitchell. "Baby Talk: The Rhetorical Production of Maternal and Fetal Selves," in *Body Talk: Rhetoric, Technology, Reproduction,* edited by Lay, Gurak, Gravon and Myntti. Madison: University of Wisconsin Press, 2000.

Granju, Kate Allison. "Formula for Disaster," www.salon.com/mwt/feature/1999/07/19/formula/, July 1999, accessed June 2005.

Gregory, Samuel. *Man-Midwifery Exposed and Corrected.* Boston: G. Gregory, 1848.

Grosz, Elizabeth. *Volatile Bodies.* New York: Routledge, 1999.

Guillemeau, Jacques. *Child-birth, or the Happy Delivery of Woman.* London, 1635.

Guttman, Nurit and Deena R. Zimmerman. "Low-Income Mothers' Views on Breastfeeding," *Social Science and Medicine* 50 no. 10, 2000: 1457–73.

Hamosh, M., et al. "Breastfeeding and the Working Mother: Effect of Time and Temperature of Short-Term storage on Proteolysis, Liposis, and Bacterial Growth in Milk," *Pediatrics* 97 no. 4, 1996: 492–98.

Haraway, Donna J. *Simians, Cyborgs and Women: The Reinvention of Nature.* New York: Routledge, 1991.

Harrison, M. R. et al. "Management of the Fetus with a Correctable Congenital Defect," *Journal of the American Medical Association* 246, 1981: 774–77.

Hartsock, Nancy. "Foucault on Power: A Theory for Women," in *Feminism/Postmodernism,* edited by Linda Nicholson. New York: Routledge, 1989.

Hausman, Bernice. *Mother's Milk: Breastfeeding Controversies in American Culture.* New York: Routledge, 2003.

Hegel, G. W. F. *Phenomenology of Spirit,* translated by A. V. Miller. New York: Oxford University Press, 1977.

Heidegger, Martin. *Being and Time,* translated by Joan Stambaugh. Albany: SUNY Press, 1996.

Hopkinson, Mrs. C. A. *Hints for the Nursery, or the Young Mother's Guide.* Boston: Little, Brown and Co., Boston, 1863.

Horowitz, Asher. *Rousseau, Nature and History.* Toronto: University of Toronto Press, 1987.

Hunter, William. *Anatomy of the Human Gravid Uterus*. Birmingham: J. Baskerville, 1774.

Irigaray, Luce. *This Sex Which Is Not One*, translated by C. Porter. Ithaca: Cornell University Press, 1995.

Ivinski, Patricia R., et al. *Farewell to the Wet-Nurse: Etienne Aubry and Images of Breast-Feeding in Eighteenth Century France*. Williamstown, MA: Sterling and Francine Clark Art Institute, 1998.

Jelliffe, D. B. and E. F. P. Jelliffe. *Human Milk in the Modern World*. Oxford: Oxford University Press, 1978.

Kaluski, D. Nitzan and A. Levinthal. "The Gift of Breastfeeding—The Practice of Breastfeeding in Israel," *Harefuah* 138 no. 8, 2000: 617–22.

Kass, Leon, with the President's Council on Bioethics. *Beyond Therapy: Biotechnology and the Pursuit of Happiness*. Washington: Regan Press, 2003.

Kearney, M. H. "Identifying Psychosocial Obstacles to Breastfeeding Success," *Journal of Obstetrical, Gynecological and Neonatal Nursing* 17 no. 2, 1988: 98–105.

Kendall-Tackett, Kathleen. "Breastfeeding and the Sexual Abuse Survivor," *Journal of Human Lactation* 14 no. 2, 1998: 125–30.

Kennel, J. H., M. A. Trause, and M. H. Klaus. "Evidence for a Sensitive Period in the Human Mother," *Ciba Foundation Symposium* 33, 1975: 87–101.

King, Helen. *Hippocrates' Women: Reading the Female Body in Ancient Greece*. New York: Routledge, 1998.

Klein, Melanie. "The Importance of Symbol-Formation in the Development of the Ego," in Volume 1 of *The Writings of Melanie Klein*, edited by R. E. Money-Kyrle et al. London: Hogarth Press, 1975.

Kneipp, Father Sebastian. *The Care of Children in Sickness and Health*, 1896. reprinted Whitefish, MT: Kessinger Publisher, 2004.

Kristeva, Julia. *Stabat Mater*, translated by A. Goldhammer, in *The Female Body in Western Culture: Contemporary Perspectives*, ed. S. Suleiman. Cambridge, MA: Harvard University Press, 1986.

Kukla, Rebecca. "Performing Nature in the Letter to M. d'Alembert," in *Rousseau on Arts and Politics: Autour de la Lettre d'Alembert*, edited by M. Butler. Ottawa: Pensées Libres, 1998: 67–77.

Kukla, Rebecca. "Talking Back: Monstrosity, Mundanity and Cynicism in Television Talk Shows," in *Rethinking Marxism* 14 no. 1, 2001: 67–96.

La Leche League International. *The Womanly Art of Breastfeeding*, Sixth Revised Edition. New York: Plume Books, 1997.

Laget, Mirelle. "Childbirth in the Seventeenth and Eighteenth Century France," in *Medicine and Society in France*, edited by R. Foster and O. Ranum. Baltimore: Johns Hopkins University Press, 1980.

Landes, Joan. *Visualizing the Nation: Gender, Representation and Revolution in Eighteenth Century France*. Ithaca: Cornell University Press, 2001.

Lauwer, Judith and Candace Woessner. *Counseling the Nursing Mother: A Reference Handbook for Health Care Providers and Lay Counselors*. Garden City Park, NY: Avery Publishing Group, 1990.

Law, Jules. "The Politics of Breastfeeding: Assessing Risk, Dividing Labour," *Signs: Journal of Women in Culture and Society* 25 no. 2, 2000: 404–50.

Lawrence, Ruth. *Breastfeeding: A Guide for the Medical Profession*, 4th edition. New York: Mosby Inc., 1994.

Lerner, Harriet E. "Effects of the Nursing Mother-Infant Dyad on the Family," *American Journal of Orthopsychiatry* 49 no. 2, 1979: 339–48.

Little, Margaret O. *Compelling Intimacy: Abortion, Law, and Morality*. Oxford University Press, Forthcoming.

Lozoff, B. "Birth and 'Bonding' in Non-Industrial Societies," *Developmental Medicine and Child Neurology* 25 no. 5, 1983: 595–600.

Lucas, A. "Breast Milk and Subsequent Intelligence Quotient in Children Born Preterm," *Lancet* 345, 1992: 261–62.

Lupton, Deborah. "Risk and the Ontology of Pregnant Embodiment," in *Risk and Sociocultural Theory*, edited by D. Lupton. New York: Cambridge University Press, 1999.

Markens, Susan, Carole H. Browner and Nancy A. Press. "Feeding the Fetus: On Interrogating the Notion of Maternal-Fetal Conflict," *Feminist Studies* 23 no. 2, 1997: 351–72.

Martin, Emily. *The Woman in the Body: A Cultural Analysis of Reproduction*. Boston: Beacon Press, 1987.

Marx, Karl. *Economic and Philosophical Manuscripts of 1844*. New York: International Publishers, 1980.

Maryland State Department of Health. *Talks to Mothers About Their Babies*. Baltimore: Bureau of Child Hygiene, 1923.

Maternity Center Association of NYC. *Maternity Handbook for Pregnant Mothers and Expectant Fathers*. New York: Putnam and Sons, 1932.

Mauquest de la Motte, Guillaume. *A General Treatise of Midwifery*. English Translation London: J. Waugh, 1746.

Mauriceau, François. *The Diseases of Women With Child and In Childbed*. Paris 1694, translated by H. Chamberlen, London: A. Bell, 1697.

Menahem, S. "Letter: Response to Fisher and Inch," *Journal of Pediatrics* 130 no. 6, 1997: 10–12.

Michaels, Meredith and Lynn Morgan, editors. *Fetal Subjects, Feminist Positions*. Philadelphia: University of Pennsylvania Press, 1999.

Michie, Helen. "Confinements: The Domestic in the Discourses of Upper-Middle Class Pregnancy," in *Making Worlds: Gender, Metaphor, Materiality*, edited by S. H. Aiken et al. Tucson, AZ: University of Arizona Press, 1998: 258–73.

Mitchell, Lisa M. and Eugenia Georges. "Cross-Cultural Cyborgs: Greek and Canadian Women's Discourses on Fetal Ultrasound," *Feminist Studies* 23 no. 2, 1997: 373–401.

Mitchell, Lisa M. *Baby's First Picture*. Toronto: University of Toronto Press, 2001.

Mitchell, Lisa M. "Women's Experiences of Unexpected Ultrasound Findings," *Journal of Midwifery and Women's Health* 49, 2004: 228–34.

Montagu, Ashley. *Touching: The Human Significance of the Skin*. New York: Columbia University Press, 1971.

Mullin, Amy. *Reconceiving Pregnancy and Childcare*. New York: Cambridge University Press, 2005.

Murkoff, H., S. Hathaway and A. Eisenberg. *What to Expect When You're Expecting*. New York: Workman Publishing, 1985/1996/2002.

Newman, Karen. *Fetal Positions*. Palo Alto: Stanford University Press, 1996.

Nash, J. Madeleine. "Inside the Womb," *Time Magazine*, November 11, 2002. Follow-up letters published December 1, 2002.

Nihell, Elizabeth. *A Treatise on the Art of Midwifery, Setting Forth Various Abuses Therein, Especially as to the Practice with Instruments*. London: A. Morely, 1760.

Oakley, Annie. *The Captured Womb: A History of the Medical Care of Pregnant Women*. London: Blackwell, 1984.

O'Neill, T., P. Murphy and V. T. Green. "Postnatal Depression—Aetiological Factors," *Irish Medical Journal* 83 no. 1, 1990: 17–18.

Orfali, Kristina. "Who Will Live? Parents Facing Ethical Dilemmas in Neonatal Intensive Care Units in France and the United States," presented at the American Society for Bioethics and the Humanities annual meeting, Montreal, October 2003.

Palmer, Gabrielle. *The Politics of Breastfeeding.* London: Pandora Press, 1988.

Papinczak, T. A. and C. T. Turner. "An Analysis of Personal and Social Factors Influencing Initiation and Duration of Breastfeeding," *Breastfeeding Review* 8 no. 1, 2000: 25–33.

Parens, Eric and Adrianne Asch, editors. *Prenatal Testing and Disability Rights.* Washington: Georgetown University Press, 2000.

Pascoe, J. M. and J. French. "The Development of Positive Feelings in Primiparous Mothers Towards Their Normal Newborns," *Clinical Pediatrics* 28 no. 10, 1989: 452–56.

Petchesky, Rosalind Pollack. "Fetal Images," *Feminist Studies* 13 no. 2, 1987: 263–76.

Petit, J. C. *Woman: Her Physical Condition, Sufferings and Maternal Relations. A Course of Parlor Lectures to Ladies,* self-published. St. Louis: 1895.

Pittard, W. B. III, et al. "Bacteriostatic Qualities of Human Milk," *Journal of Pediatrics* 107 no. 2, 1985: 240–43.

Pittard W. B. III, et al. "Bacterial Contamination of Human milk: Container Type and Method of Expression," *American Journal of Perinatology* 8 no. 1, 1991: 25–27.

Plato. *Timeus,* translated by Donald J. Zeyl. Indianapolis: Hackett, 2000.

Pollit, Katha. "'Fetal Rights': A New Assault on Feminism," in *'Bad' Mothers: The Politics of Blame in Twentieth Century America,* edited by R. Ladd-Taylor and P. Umansky. New York: New York University Press, 1998.

Portal, Paul. *The Complete Practice of Men and Women Midwives, or, The True Manner of Assisting a Woman in Child-Bearing.* trans. London: H. Clark, 1705.

Pridham, K. E. et al. "The Relation of a Mother's Working Model of Feeding to Her Feeding Behaviour," *Journal of Advanced Nursing* 35 no. 5, 2001: 741–50.

Quant, Sara. "Sociocultural Aspects of the Lactation Process," in *Breastfeeding: Biocultural Perspectives,* edited by P. Stuart-MacAdam and K. A. Dettwyler. New York: De Gruyter, 1995.

Rapp, Rayna. *Testing Women, Testing the Fetus.* New York: Routledge, 1999.

Riordan, J. M. and E. T. Rapp. "Pleasure and Purpose: The Sensuousness of Breastfeeding," *Journal of Obstetric and Gynecological Neonatal Nursing* 9 no. 2, 1980: 109–12.

Robin, Peggy. *Bottlefeeding Without Guilt: A Reassuring Guide for Loving Parents.* Rocklin, CA: Prima Publishing, 1995.

Rodriguez-Garcia, R and L. Frazier. "Cultural Paradoxes Relating to Sexuality and Breastfeeding," *Journal of Human Lactation* 11 no. 2, 1995: 111–15.

Rogers, J. S., J. Golding and P. M. Emmett. "The Effects of Lactation on the Mother," *Early Human Development* 49 supplement, 1997: 191–203.

Rothman, Barbara Katz. *The Tentative Pregnancy: How Amniocentesis Changes the Experience of Motherhood.* New York: Norton, 1993.

Rousseau, Jean-Jacques. *Confessions,* translated by J. M. Cohen. New York: Penguin, 1953.

Rousseau, Jean-Jacques. *Oeuvres Completes de Jean-Jacques Rousseau,* edited by B. Gagnebin and M. Raymond. Paris: Gallimard, Biblotèque de Pléiade, 1959.

Rousseau, Jean-Jacques. *Julie, ou la Nouvelle Heloïse.* Paris: Editions Garnier Frères, 1961.

Rousseau, Jean-Jacques. "Letter to d'Alembert," reprinted in *Politics and the Arts,* translated by A. Bloom. Ithaca: Cornell University Press, 1968.

Rousseau, Jean-Jacques. *Emile, or On Education,* translated by A. Bloom. New York: Basic Books, 1979.

Rousseau, Jean-Jacques. *Reveries of a Solitary Walker*, translated by P. France. London: Penguin, 1979.

Rousseau, Jean-Jacques. *The Government of Poland*, translated by Willmore Kendall. Indianapolis: Hackett, 1985.

Rousseau, Jean-Jacques. *On the Social Contract*, translated by Donald A. Cress. Indianapolis: Hackett, 1987.

Rousseau, Jean-Jacques. *The Collected Writings of Rousseau*, translated and edited by R. Masters and C. Kelly. Hanover, NH: University Press of New England, 1990.

Rousseau, Jean-Jacques. *Discourse on the Origins of Inequality*, trans. Donald A. Cress. Indianapolis: Hackett, 1992.

Roussillon, J. A. "Adult Survivors of Sexual Abuse: Suggestions for Perinatal Caregivers," *Clinical Excellence for Nurse Practitioners* 2 no. 6, 1998: 329–37.

Ruddick, Sara. *Maternal Thinking: Towards a Politics of Peace*. Boston: Beacon Press, 1989.

Rüff, Jakob. *De Conceptu et Generatione Hominus*. Francofurti ad Moenum: Christophorus Froscho, 1554 (translated London 1637).

Sade, Marquis de. *Philosophie Dans le Boudoir*, translated and reprinted in *Justine, Philosophy in the Bedroom, and Other Stories*. New York: Grove Press, 1990.

Sadler, John. *The Sicke Woman's Private Looking-Glasse*. 1636, reprinted London: Theatrum Orbis, 1977.

Sartre, Jean-Paul. *Existentialism and Human Emotions*. New York: Philosophical Library, 1957.

Scheman, Naomi. "Anger and the Politics of Naming," in *Engenderings*, New York: Routledge, 1993.

Seema-Patwary, A. K. and L. Satyanarayana. "Relactation: An Effective Intervention to Promote Exclusive Breastfeeding," *Journal of Tropical Pediatrics* 43 no. 4, 1997: 213–16.

Seigel, Marika. "Visualizing and Individualizing Risk During Pregnancy," presented at the Society for Literature and Science meeting, Durham, NC, October 2004.

Sermon, William. *The Ladies' companion, or the English Midwife, wherein is demonstrated the manner and order how women ought to govern themselves during the whole times of their breeding children and of their difficult labour, hard travail, and lying-in. etc., together with the diseases they are subject to, especially in such times and the several wayes and means to help them; also the various forms of the child's proceeding forth of the womb, in 17 copper cuts, with a discourse of the parts principally serving for generation*. London: Edward Thomas, 1671.

Sharp, Jane. *The Midwives Book, or, the Whole Art of Midwifery Discovered*. 1671, reprinted New York: Oxford University Press, 1999.

Shelley, Mary. *Frankenstein, or, the Modern Prometheus*. London: H. Colburn and R. Bentley, 1831.

Shildrick, Margrit. *Leaky Bodies and Boundaries*. New York: Routledge, 1997.

Shildrick, Margrit. *Embodying the Monster: Encounters with the Vulnerable Self*. Thousand Oaks: Sage Publications, 2002.

Simms, Eva-Marie. "Milk and Flesh: A Phenomenological Reflection on Infancy and Coexistence," *Journal of Phenomenological Psychology*, 32 no. 1, 2001: 22–40.

Smellie, William. *A Treatise on the Theory and Practice of Midwifery*, in 3 volumes. London: D. Wilson, 1752.

Smellie, William. *A Set of Anatomical Tables, with Explanations, and an Abridgment, of the Practice of Midwifery, With a View to Illustrate a Treatise on That Subject, and a Collection of Cases*. London: 1754.

Smith, Mark Eddy. "Nursing the World Back to Health," *New Beginnings* 12 no. 3, 1995: 68–71.

Squier, Susan. "Fetal Subjects and Maternal Objects: Reproductive Technology and the New Fetal/Maternal Relation," *Journal of Medicine and Philosophy*, 21 no. 5, 1996: 515–35.

Speert, Harold. *Obstetric and Gynecologic Milestones Illustrated*. New York: Parthenon Publishing Group, 1996.

Spock, Benjamin. *Dr. Spock's Baby and Child Care*, 8th edition. New York: Pocket, 2004.

Stevenson, Roger. *The Fetus and Newly Born Infant: Influences of the Prenatal Environment*. St. Louis: Mosby, 1973.

Sussman, George. *Selling Mothers' Milk: The Wet-Nursing Business in France*. Urbana: University of Illinois Press, 1982.

Tamaro, Janet. *So That's What They're For! Breastfeeding Basics*. Holbrook, MA: Adams Media, 1998.

Taylor, Janelle. "The Public Fetus and the Family Car: From Abortion Politics to a Volvo Advertisement," *Public Culture* 4 no. 2, 1992: 67–79.

Terry, Jennifer. "The Body Invaded: Medical Surveillance of Women as Reproducers," *Socialist Review* 19, 1989: 13–43.

Thicknesse, Philip. *Man-Midwifery Analyzed*. London: R. Davis, 1764.

Thompson, Judith Jarvis. "A Defense of Abortion," *Philosophy and Public Affairs* 1 no. 1, 1971: 47–66.

Timor-Tritsch, I. E. and L. D. Platt. "Three-Dimensional Ultrasound Experience in Obstetrics," *Current Opinion in Obstetrics and Gynecology*, 14 no. 6, 2002: 569–75.

Traina, C. "Passionate Mothering: Toward an Ethic of Appropriate Mother-Child Intimacy," *Annual of the Society of Christian Ethics*, 18, 1998: 177–96.

Tsiaris, Alexander. *From Conception to Birth: A Life Unfolds*. New York: Doubleday, 2002.

Turner, Daniel. *The Force of the Mother's Imagination upon her Fetus in Utero*. London: J. Walthoe, 1730.

Ummarino, M. et al. "Short Duration of Breastfeeding and Early Introduction of Breast-Milk as a Result of Mothers' Low Level of Education," *Acta Paediactrica* 92, 2003: 12–17.

United States Department of Labor Children's Bureau. *Infant Care*. Washington, DC: Government Printing Office, 1926.

United States Department of Health and Human Services. "Public Health Campaign to Promote Breastfeeding Awareness Launched," Press Release June 2004, www.hhs.gov/news/press/2004pres/20040604.html, accessed June 2005.

United States Department of Health and Human Services. "Education Campaign Takes on Lagging Breastfeeding Rates: Few Babies Breastfed Long Enough," *The Nation's Health* 34 no. 7, September 2004: 4–5.

Uvnas-Moberg, K. and Eriksson, M. "Breastfeeding: Physiological, Endocrine and Behavioral Adaptations Caused by Oxytocin and Local Neurogenic Activity in the Nipple and Mammary Gland," *Acta Paediatrica*, 85 no. 5, 1996: 525–30.

Valdes, V. et al. "Clinical Support Can Make the Difference in Exclusive Breastfeeding Success Among Working Women," *Journal of Tropical Pediatrics* 46 no. 3, 2000: 149–54.

Van Blarcom, Carolyn C., R. N. *Getting Ready To Be A Mother*. New York: Macmillan, 1932.

Walker, Michele Boulos. *Philosophy and the Maternal Body: Reading Silence*. New York: Routledge, 1998.

Ward, Julie D. *La Leche League: At the Crossroads of Medicine, Feminism and Religion.* Chapel Hill: University of North Carolina Press, 2000.

Weir, Lorna. "Pregnancy Ultrasound in Maternal Discourse," in *Vital Signs: Feminist Reconfigurations of the Bio/Logical Body*, edited by Margrit Shildrick and Janet Price. Edinburgh: Edinburgh University Press, 1998.

Wells, H. G. *The Island of Dr. Moreau*, edited by R. M. Philmus. Athens, GA: University of Georgia Press, 1896/1993.

White, Charles. *A Treatise on the Management of Pregnant and Lying-In Women.* 1773, London, reprinted by Canton, MA: Science History Publications, 1987.

Williams, Al-Yasha Ilhaam and Ina May Gaskin, "Elective Cesareans as Reproductive Choice: Some Ethical Considerations," unpublished manuscript, 2004.

Williams, Nancy. "Maternal Psychological Issues in the Experience of Breastfeeding," *Journal of Human Lactation* 13 no. 1, 1997: 57–60.

Winnicott, D. W. *The Child and the Family.* London: Tavistock, 1958.

Wolf, Naomi. *Misconceptions: Truth, Lies and the Unexpected on the Journey to Motherhood.* New York: Doubleday Books, 2001.

Yalom, Miriam. *A History of the Breast.* New York: Ballantine Books, 1997.

Young, Iris. "Pregnant Embodiment: Subjectivity and Alienation," *Journal of Medicine and Philosophy* 9, 1984: 45–62.

Zerilli, Linda. *Signifying Woman: Culture and Chaos in Rousseau, Burke, and Mill.* Ithaca: Cornell University Press, 1994.

Zizek, Slavoj. *The Sublime Object of Ideology.* New York: Verso, 1989.

Zizek, Slavoj. "Kant and Sade: The Ideal Couple," *lacanian ink* 13, http://www.lacan.com/frameXIII2.htm, 2001, accessed June 2005.

Index

2001: A Space Odyssey, 111
abortion, 4, 109, 111, 117
accoucheurs. *See* midwifery, man-midwifery
American Academy of Pediatrics (AAP), 145, 158, 161, 170–71, 204, 208
American Revolution, 34
appetites: during pregnancy, 6, 11, 12, 13–19, 21, 69, 83, 84, 85, 88, 106–7, 118–19, 218; of man-midwives, 88; sexual, 69, 83–85, 88, 106–7, 118–19, 218; of the uterus, 5, 12, 13, 118. *See also* maternal imagination, theory of; passions
artificial milk. *See* infant formula
Ashley, Kawana, 122
attachment theory/ "attachment parenting," 145, 150, 168–69, 174, 182n35. *See also* proximity (as principle of good mothering)
authority over maternal bodies: medical, 18, 71–72, 85, 127–35, 171–75, 218; social, 17–18, 49, 66–67, 70, 83–88, 127–35, 136, 218, 219, 226

birth, 8, 21, 25n3, 59, 72, 78, 86–92, 108, 133–34, 173, 219, 222–24; cesarean section, 173, 222, 233n8; fetal monitoring during, 107–8; instrument use during, 8, 73, 78, 87–91, 219; "natural" childbirth, 21, 59, 88–91, 219, 222–24

birth defects, 6, 8, 9, 10, 11, 13–19, 21, 22, 23, 50, 70, 78, 87, 105, 126, 131. *See also* Down syndrome; prenatal testing; maternal imagination, theory of; monsters/monstrosity
Blum, Linda, 150, 156–59, 228
Blunt, John, 86, 87, *90*, 90–91
bonding, maternal, 30, 49, 112–20, 148–52, 167, 168–71, 175, 183n57, 185nn84–85, 222; during breastfeeding, 30, 49, 148–49, 150–52, 167, 168–71, 175, 183n57, 185nn84–85; with fetus, 112–20; ultrasound imaging and, 117–18. *See also* breastmilk as bond between mother and child; Harlow monkey experiments
bottle feeding. *See* bottles/artificial feeders
bottles/artificial feeders, 152–53, 154, 158–59, 160–63, 164–65, 169–70, 171–72, 174, 198, 226. *See also* breastfeeding; breastmilk, expressed; infant formula; nipples, artificial
breastfeeding, 30–34, 42–53, 56–57, 66, 68, 80, 93–97, 145–75, 190–213, 223, 225; advocacy campaigns, 145–46, 192–93, 211; "babies were born to be breastfed" campaign, 145–46, *190*, 192–93, 211; barriers to, 192–96, 200–1, 209; discomfort during, 190–91, 193–96, 202–4, 212; health

About the Author

Rebecca Kukla is an associate professor of philosophy at Carleton University in Ottawa, Canada, as well as an affiliated associate professor at the Kennedy Institute of Ethics at Georgetown University. From 2003–2005, she was a Greenwall Fellow in Bioethics and Health Policy at Johns Hopkins University. She is the editor of *Aesthetics and Cognition in Kant's Critical Philosophy* (forthcoming, 2006), as well as the author of numerous articles and book chapters on ethics, epistemology, philosophy of science and medicine, eighteenth-century philosophy, and feminist theory.